ILLUMINATED
HEALING

Unraveling The Mysteries
Of Light Therapy

DR. CARL ROTHSCHILD, D.C.

Important Information For the Reader

The content in this book is derived from my personal experiences and comprehensive research, focusing on the subject of light therapy. This book should not be used for self-diagnosis or as a self-treatment guide, nor should it replace the advice and attention given by a licensed health care provider. It is strongly encouraged to discuss the information gleaned from this book with your primary care physician.

This book aims to guide you in making informed decisions about your long-term health targets. If you find yourself dealing with any health issues, it is critical that you immediately consult with a professional health care practitioner. Keep in mind, early assessment and detection play a crucial role in successfully managing any health condition.

TABLE OF CONTENTS

An Introduction To Red Light Therapy...1

Chapter 1: The History Of Red Light Therapy 14

Chapter 2: How RLT Physically And Biochemically
Affects The Body..35

Chapter 3: The Science Behind Red Light Therapy 50

Chapter 4: Some Of The Red Light Therapy Devices Available . 66

Chapter 5: How RLT May Support Anti-Aging.........................73

Chapter 6: Red Light Therapy And Cellular Health.................82

Chapter 7: Cellular Energy And RLT 98

Chapter 8: Red Light Therapy And Pain Relief......................108

Chapter 9: Skin Health And The Benefits Of RLT 120

Chapter 10: Red Light Therapy And Muscle Recovery...........129

Chapter 11: RLT And Weight Loss..141

Chapter 12: Joint Health And Red Light Therapy 152

Chapter 13: Red Light Therapy And Hormonal Health...........164

Chapter 14: Brain Function And RLT.....................................175

Chapter 15: Red Light Therapy And Inflammation.................188

Chapter 16: Telomere Health And RLT 201

Chapter 17: Immune Function And Red Light Therapy.........214

Chapter 18: Red Light Therapy And Detoxification 223

Chapter 19: Lifestyle Modifications Which May Enhance RLT 234

Chapter 20: Choosing The Right Red Light Therapy Provider 247

Chapter 21: The Incredible Power And Benefits Of
Red Light Therapy 255

AN INTRODUCTION TO
RED LIGHT THERAPY

As a devoted chiropractor with over four decades of experience, my intention has been to promote and innovate efficient methods that offer rapid and effective relief for patients. It is with great pride that I present the Trifecta Light Bed to you. This is a cutting-edge device, conceived through my dedication to patient care and the culmination of years of rigorous research and development. In this book, I will impart my personal insights and expertise on the revolutionary technology of red light therapy. As a practitioner, you will acquire an in-depth comprehension of this therapy's numerous health benefits, which will enable you to make well-informed decisions regarding its implementation and power.

My qualifications emanate from institutions such as Stony Brook University and the Los Angeles College of Chiropractic, as well as my role as the director of the Westland Health Center and my status as a diplomate of the National Board of Chiropractic Examiners. These accomplishments have uniquely positioned me to make significant contributions to the field of red light therapy, and the Trifecta Light Bed stands as a testament to this therapy's proven efficacy in addressing many health concerns.

From headaches, back and neck pain, muscle pain, allergies, and sports injuries, to automobile and work injuries, this versatile and potent device proves invaluable in the hands of adept practitioners. As you explore this book, I aim to convey the technological wonder of red light therapy and impart my fervor for public health and safety. Throughout my career, I have actively participated in numerous public speaking events in the Los Angeles area, educating and informing countless individuals on ergonomics and other essential health issues. Under my guidance, you will harness the remarkable potential benefits of Red Light Therapy and possibly transform the lives of those seeking relief from pain and discomfort.

I invite you to embrace the future of healthcare with red light therapy and to join me in enhancing the well-being of patients worldwide. In recent years, red light therapy (also known as "RLT") has gained immense popularity due to its non-invasive nature, which employs red and near-infrared light to stimulate cellular activity within the body. This therapy elicits various health benefits by initiating specific biochemical reactions that ultimately restore cellular function. RLT has demonstrated an extensive range of potential applications across diverse fields of medicine and wellness, and its utilization continues to expand.

For instance, it has been found to improve skin health by reducing inflammation and promoting collagen production, resulting in enhanced skin texture and tone and a diminished appearance of fine lines and wrinkles. According to a study by Leanne Venier in 2017, published in the Journal of Optics and Photonics, red light therapy has demonstrated the potential to alleviate pain and reduce inflammation in patients suffering from chronic pain conditions such as osteoarthritis, TMJ, and fibromyalgia. The study revealed that RLT can decrease pain levels by up to 60%, with results lasting up to one-month post-treatment.

Indeed, this promising therapy exhibits immense potential in optimizing cellular function, fostering healing, mitigating inflammation, and assuaging pain, all of which make it a powerful tool for fostering good health and supporting healing.

Red Light Therapy

Light has a long history of being used as a therapeutic tool since the ancient Greeks who used sunlight and sunbathing for various ailments. The therapeutic potential of red light was discovered further in the 1960s by NASA scientists searching for ways to help astronauts heal injuries and maintain optimal health in space. Red light, at specific wavelengths, was found to increase the rate of tissue repair and reduce inflammation in the body. Numerous studies have since then been carried out to explore the additional benefits of red light therapy, including the treatment of chronic pain, its anti-aging properties, and in regard to musculoskeletal disorders.

Red Light Therapy, or "RLT" for short, is a term we use to indicate both Red Light and Near-Infrared wavelengths. It involves using LEDs that emit light within a range of 600-1000 nanometers (nm). Red light is absorbed by the body, stimulating cell energy production and promoting tissue regeneration. Near-infrared light goes deeper into the body, reaching muscles, bones, and joints, which can help with healing and reduce inflammation.

In short, red light therapy in essence works by increasing ATP production, which is the energy currency of cells. This enhances cellular function and promotes healing at a cellular level. Although not all devices are created equally, the dosage, wavelength, and duration of exposure determines the effectiveness of the therapy. Weaker devices are not potent enough to produce any remarkable benefits. Red light therapy, also called "Photobiomodulation," or PBM for short, has transformed the medical industry over the last decades. By applying light energy to the skin, light penetrates the body's tissue and is absorbed by cells, leading to improved mitochondrial function and enhanced cellular energy production. This heightened energy production, in turn, leads to numerous benefits regarding physical and emotional well-being. Light therapy devices are classified into four distinct classes, by the Food and Drug Administration (FDA), with Class 1 and 2 being devices that are available for anyone to purchase. In contrast, Class 3 and 4 devices, which include Laser and Intense Pulsed Light equipment, require a professional license before use.

Throughout the years, red light therapy has been the subject of extensive scientific research, which has revealed its vast benefits. It is considered a non-invasive and safe therapy. Over the years, this therapeutic approach has gained considerable attention for its wide range of applications, which now includes nerve pain relief for patients suffering from neuropathy, anti-aging treatments in spas, weight loss support in various health clinics, as an adjunct therapy to support good mental health, in the reduction of inflammation, and as part of protocols for diabetic wound care and healing.

In the context of nerve pain associated with neuropathy, red light therapy has been known to improve nerve function, reduce inflammation, and alleviate neuropathic pain. The therapy targets the affected nerves by emitting light energy, which is then absorbed by the cellular structures. As already mentioned, this process, in turn, enhances the production of ATP and stimulates the release of nitric oxide, which is a potent vasodilator. Consequently, blood circulation, oxygenation, and nutrient delivery to the damaged nerves improve, thereby promoting regeneration and reducing neuropathic pain. Red light therapy has now also been incorporated into many anti-aging spa treatments to address common skin concerns such as wrinkles, fine lines, blemishes and age spots. Red light therapy has been shown to stimulate collagen and elastin production within the skin, two essential proteins responsible for maintaining the skin's elasticity and firmness. Additionally, it aids in reducing inflammation and promoting cellular repair, which can contribute to a healthier, more youthful complexion.

Furthermore, weight loss modalities have begun to explore the potential benefits of red light therapy in facilitating fat reduction. The therapy is believed to affect adipocytes, or the fat-storing cells, by prompting the release of stored lipids which are then metabolized by the body for energy. This process, combined with exercise and a balanced diet, can support weight loss efforts and help individuals achieve their desired body composition. On the other side of the spectrum of care, mental health is another area where red light therapy has shown great promise. The therapy is thought to influence the production of neurotransmitters such as serotonin and dopamine, which play a crucial role in mood regulation. By modulating these chemical messengers, red light therapy has been shown to be able to help alleviate symptoms of depression, anxiety, and other mental health disorders.

Furthermore, red light therapy has been linked to improved cognitive function and enhanced sleep quality, both of which contribute to overall mental well-being. Additionally, chronic inflammation is a common denominator in many chronic health conditions and autoimmune disorders, such as Rheumatoid arthritis, and the symptoms relayed to many of these conditions may also be alleviated through red light therapy. Red light has been known to reduce inflammation by promoting the release of anti-inflammatory compounds while inhibiting the production of pro-inflammatory cytokines. This process has not only been shown to be able to alleviate the pain and discomfort associated with inflammation, but also supports the body's natural healing processes.

Red light therapy has additionally demonstrated its effectiveness in the treatment of non-healing diabetic wounds. Wound healing in individuals with diabetes can be very challenging due to impaired blood circulation and persistent inflammation, and in some cases becomes impossible to manage and, in the end, may lead to amputation. Red light therapy, however, has been shown to be able to address this issue by promoting blood flow, reducing inflammation, and stimulating cellular repair and angiogenesis (the creation of new blood vessels). Consequently, diabetic wounds treated with red light therapy may exhibit accelerated healing rates and a lowered risk of complications.

In conclusion, red light therapy has emerged as a versatile and promising treatment modality for various health concerns. It holds great promise as an adjunct therapy for many existing modalities and treatments. By its non-invasive nature, coupled with its proven ability to target a wide range of issues, it can be argued to be an attractive option for individuals who seek a safe and effective therapeutic intervention. As additional scientific research is conducted, the full potential of red light therapy continues to be discovered, and its application will, without question, become more widely implemented in the medical field as an effective and highly technical therapeutic option.

The Different Types Of
Red Light Therapy

As already mentioned, RLT utilizes light-emitting diodes (or LEDs) to deliver therapeutic benefits to the body in a non-invasive manner. By targeting different wavelengths of light to penetrate the skin's layers, along with the muscles and joints, it has been found to offer a wide range of health benefits. LLLT employs a focused beam of light to directly deliver specific wavelengths of light to individual cells within the body, and LLLT has been shown to be highly effective in treating chronic pain, reducing inflammation, promoting wound healing, renewed hair growth, and improving an array of skin conditions, such as acne and psoriasis, as well as reducing many classical signs of aging through its ability to enhance collagen production. On the other hand, LED therapy employs a broad-spectrum approach that targets larger areas of the body with a wide range of wavelengths. The process activates the cells within the skin's dermis, which in turn has been found to lead to a decrease in inflammation and pain. LED therapy has shown great promise as an effective treatment option for arthritis, postoperative pain, and various skin conditions, including rosacea and acne. It has also been shown to be able to enhance immune function and promote new hair growth.

The science behind RLT's technical advances has become a topic of increasing interest among the medical community and the general public. The technique's ability to promote healing and reduce pain and inflammation, combined with its non-invasive nature, has opened the door for many new possibilities to promote healing and alleviate discomfort within various conditions. As we learn more about how different wavelengths of light may impact the body, we can look forward to further discoveries and developments in this groundbreaking technique.

The Evolution of Red Light Therapy Over Time

The origins of Red Light Therapy (RLT) can be traced back to the late 1960s when NASA began researching the effects of light on plant growth. NASA scientists discovered that red light could effectively enhance the growth and development of plants by increasing their photosynthetic capacity. Further research then led to the discovery that red light could also positively affect human cells. In the early 1990s, RLT was first used in clinical trials to treat non-healing wounds caused by diabetes. The trials revealed that RLT could accelerate the healing process and improve the quality of life for patients. Consequently, RLT began gaining recognition in the medical field.

In the following years, research on the therapeutic benefits of RLT continued, ultimately leading to its effectiveness in treating a range of conditions, such as chronic pain, arthritis, and depression. Further research discoveries have led to new uses of RLT in sports medicine for muscle recovery and for conditions like acne and psoriasis in dermatology. NASA has played an essential role in the origins of RLT by undertaking the initial research into the benefits of light on the human body. The research provided a foundation for further discoveries that have contributed to the advancement of RLT's therapeutic applications, transforming it into a vital and innovative therapy used by a range of medical professionals today. RLT quickly emerged as a vital treatment option once its potential benefits became evident. According to a study conducted by Hamblin et al. (2010), RLT has shown promising outcomes in the early stages of medical application. The study revealed that RLT promoted wound healing in skin injuries such as burns and diabetic ulcers. Owing to these discoveries, RLT has become ubiquitous in dermatology, serving as a vital tool in the industry. Similarly, RLT found promise in treating musculoskeletal injuries, particularly among athletes. Consequently, sports medicine practitioners began utilizing RLT to alleviate pain and inflammation, and promote the healing of soft tissues such as muscles, tendons, and ligaments.

As medical professionals began using RLT more frequently, the technology behind this treatment method improved drastically. Initially, RLT involved the use of large and bulky machines that only emitted red light at certain and very specific wavelengths. However, technological advancement led to the evolution of smaller and more portable devices, like the hand-held devices, light beds, and panels we now have today.

Recent advancements in technology have exponentially expanded RLT's range of applications. For instance, RLT has now also been shown to be able to assist in dental procedures and neurologically-based treatments. In 2019, researchers from the School and Hospital of Stomatology at Wuhan University in China conducted a meta-analysis study titled "Effectiveness of Low-Level Laser Therapy in the Management of Orthodontic Pain," published in the journal Photobiomodulation, Photomedicine, and Laser Surgery. The study examined data from 14 randomized controlled trials that explored using RLT to diminish orthodontic pain. According to the results, RLT greatly reduced pain levels and improved patient-reported outcomes compared to other methods, such as placebo or control treatments. The authors believe that RLT is a safe and effective choice for managing discomfort and pain associated with orthodontics. As technology continues to develop, we will likely continue to uncover new applications and utilizations for RLT to promote patient health and vitality.

Recent scientific literature demonstrates RLT as both very safe and effective. As studies suggest RLT's potential to also enhance cognitive function, memory, and attention span and alleviate symptoms of depression, we may yet witness a wider development of its therapeutic benefits. In 2020, a study was conducted by researchers from the University of São Paulo, Brazil, and published in the journal Frontiers in Neuroscience. The study, titled "Acute Effects of Light Emitting Diodes Therapy (LEDT) on Cognition and Mood in Healthy Young Adults: A Randomized, Double-Blind, Placebo-Controlled Crossover Trial," examined the effects of Red Light Therapy (RLT) on cognitive function and mood in healthy young adults. In the study, participants were randomly assigned to either red light or placebo light for 20 minutes. After that, their cognitive function and mood were measured using standardized tests. The findings revealed that those exposed to red light had better cognitive function, attention span, and memory performance compared to those exposed to placebo light. The authors believe that the reason for these positive effects could be attributed to the boost in cerebral blood flow and improved mitochondrial function in the brain.

Trifecta Light stands as a leading provider and distributor of full-body red light therapy systems, and our focus is on supplying advanced technology that may offer numerous potential benefits, such as skin rejuvenation and overall promoted healing. Our device has gained widespread recognition from healthcare professionals and wellness facilities, elevating their services significantly. With red light therapy, nearly everyone can now seek out an effective method to enhance their physical well-being, and the Trifecta stands as one of the most advanced red light therapy devices available today. I sincerely hope that I have succeeded in illuminating the many facets of red light therapy and, more specifically, the technological strides embodied in the creation of the Trifecta Light Bed. As its developer, my objective surpasses mere technological advancement. I aim to redefine and improve health and wellness by making strides toward a future where chronic ailments find no foothold and where patients may recover from ill health by natural and non-invasive means.

This device, with its profound potential, is the embodiment of countless hours of research and development. It is the fruit of an unwavering commitment to provide a therapeutic solution that is non-invasive yet remarkably effective! The science is sound and the results are real. Yet, it is essential to bear in mind that as with any scientific discovery, understanding is key. The aim of this book is not just to showcase the Trifecta and its possibilities but to truly enlighten you about the nuanced science that embodies this therapy.

We are embarking on a journey of knowledge together, and it is one I hope you will find just as fascinating as I do.

As you read further, you will be enlightened on the biology, the research, and the transformative impact of this therapy. May this book serve as a comprehensive guide and a resource that empowers you to make an informed decision about the health and well-being of your patients and clients. It is my honor to share my knowledge of this powerful therapy with you, and I am confident that, by reading this book, you will come to appreciate not just the ingenuity of this technology but also the profound benefits that it brings to the future of our healthcare. Together, let us step into the light of a healthier, brighter future!

CHAPTER 1

THE HISTORY OF RED
LIGHT THERAPY

As we delve into the fascinating world of red light therapy, it is important to understand the history behind this revolutionary form of treatment. This technology has come a long way since its early beginnings as a treatment for chronic pain and inflammation. In this chapter, I wish to elaborate on its rich history and emphasize the many technological advancements that have revolutionized this therapeutic modality and which have led to the development of many innovative devices, such as the Trifecta Light Bed.

From the initial discovery of the therapeutic effects of red light by Niels Ryberg Finsen in the late 19th century to the advent of low-level laser therapy (LLLT) in the 1960s, and the emergence of the light-emitting diode (LED) technology in recent years, red light therapy has undergone a remarkable transformation. As scientific understanding of the biological and physiological effects of red light has grown, so too has the range of conditions that may be affected and benefit from this incredible technology, from skin rejuvenation to wound healing and even cognitive enhancement.

Throughout its history, some pivotal moments have shaped the evolution of red light therapy through the contributions of pioneering researchers and clinicians who have dedicated their careers to advancing our knowledge of this powerful healing modality. I intend to offer you a deeper appreciation for the history and potential of red light therapy and the exciting possibilities that lie ahead as we continue to push the boundaries of this life-changing technology.

The Power Of Sunlight

The use of light in healing practices dates back to ancient civilizations, with historical records showing that various cultures utilized sunlight exposure and heliotherapy for therapeutic purposes. From the ancient and traditional usage of heliotherapy and sunlight exposure, many early practices laid the foundation for the development of the modern red light therapy we know today.

The ancient Egyptians were among the first to recognize the healing power of sunlight! They practiced a specific healing modality called "heliotherapy," which is the therapeutic use of sunlight, and utilized sunbaths to treat various ailments, such as skin diseases, joint disorders, and nervous system conditions. In addition to sunlight therapy, the Egyptians were also known to use colored glass and gemstones in the attempt to harness the therapeutic effects of different light wavelengths. This concept is echoed in the technology behind the modern Trifecta Light Bed.

The renowned Greek physician Hippocrates, often referred to as the "Father of Medicine," was also an advocate for sunlight exposure as a means of promoting health and wellness. He recommended that patients with tuberculosis (which is a disease that affects the lungs and can cause severe respiratory problems) should be exposed to sunlight to help alleviate their symptoms. Hippocrates also believed that sunlight exposure could help treat various other health issues, such as depression and insomnia, by promoting the production of mood-enhancing chemicals in the brain. Traditional Chinese Medicine (abbreviated to TCM) has long incorporated the use of sunlight in its healing practices.

The philosophy and medical system of Chinese medicine are built upon the Five Elements Theory – Wood, Fire, Earth, Metal, and Water are thought to be the fundamental building blocks of the universe. In this philosophy, sunlight is associated with the Fire element, which is, in turn, considered to be a vital life force that sustains and nourishes the body. In TCM, sunlight exposure is often prescribed to help balance the body's energy and improve overall health, with specific times of the day and body positions designated for optimal sunbathing practices.

This age-old concept of harnessing the sun's energy is, in effect, mirrored in the design of the Trifecta Light Bed, which uses the power of red light therapy to stimulate the body's natural healing processes.

Ayurveda, the ancient Indian system of medicine, also incorporates sunlight exposure as a healing practice. Ayurvedic teachings assert that the sun is a powerful source of energy and life and that regular sunlight exposure is essential for maintaining physical, mental, and spiritual well-being. Ayurvedic practitioners often recommend sunbathing during specific times, such as early morning or late afternoon, when the sun's rays are considered most beneficial for health. Additionally, they may incorporate the use of natural oils and herbs to enhance the therapeutic effects of sunlight on the skin and body. Throughout the history of Man, the ancient and traditional use of heliotherapy and sunlight exposure in various cultures around the world highlights the powerful healing potential of light. These early practices laid the groundwork for the development of modern light therapy techniques, such as the red light therapy employed by the Trifecta Light Bed.

By understanding the historical context and cultural significance of light therapy, we may better appreciate the innovative technology that enables us to harness the healing power of light in a safe, effective, and accessible manner.

The Pioneers of Phototherapy

As we delve into the history of red light therapy, we would not do this incredible technology justice without recognizing the first pioneers of phototherapy, who essentially paved the way for the development and innovations that have led to the red light therapy we know today. Phototherapy, or simply "light therapy," exposes the skin and body to bright ultraviolet (UV) rays for its believed healing benefits. These early trailblazers include Niels Ryberg Finsen, Auguste and Louis Lumière, and John Harvey Kellogg, who each contributed significantly to our current understanding of the therapeutic effects of light wavelengths and their applications in medicine.

Niels Ryberg Finsen

Niels Ryberg Finsen was a Danish physician and scientist and is considered one of the founding figures in the field of phototherapy. In the late 19th century, Finsen developed "the Finsen Light," which is a powerful carbon arc lamp that produced ultraviolet light. His invention was inspired by his observation that sunlight had a positive impact on various skin conditions, which led Finsen to explore the therapeutic potential of different light wavelengths - particularly ultraviolet light, which he believed could have bactericidal effects and promote wound healing.

In 1903, Finsen was awarded the Nobel Prize in Medicine for his groundbreaking work in treating lupus vulgaris, a disfiguring skin disease caused by tuberculosis bacteria, with ultraviolet light. Finsen's successful treatment of lupus patients with his Finsen Light demonstrated the potential of light therapy in medicine and laid the foundation for future research in phototherapy.

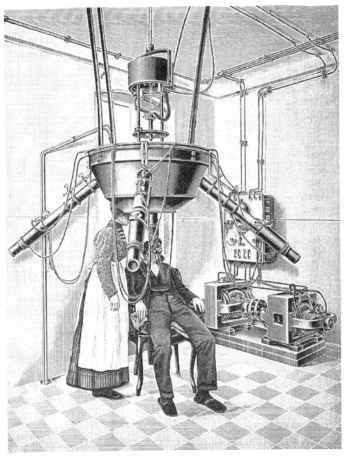

The Finsen Light, 1902, from the Contributing Library
of Francis A. Countway Library of Medicine.

Another pair of early pioneers in phototherapy were the French inventors and filmmakers Auguste and Louis Lumière. The Lumière brothers, best known for their development of the motion picture camera, were also fascinated with the therapeutic effects of light. Their early research focused on the potential benefits of different light wavelengths, and they were among the first to recognize the healing properties of red and infrared light. The Lumière brothers' investigations into the therapeutic effects of light helped to broaden our understanding of the potential applications of phototherapy in medicine.

Additionally, John Harvey Kellogg, who was an American physician and inventor, was another important figure in the early development of phototherapy. Mr. Kellogg, who is perhaps best known as the co-inventor of cornflakes, was also an advocate of natural remedies and believed in the power of light to promote health and well-being. In the early 1900s, Kellogg invented the "incandescent light bath," which was a device that exposed the body to intense light and heat from incandescent lamps. The person would be seated in a sauna-like, enclosed space, surrounded by and bathed in light. The first incandescent light bath was invented in 1891, and Kellogg believed that the light and heat from the incandescent lamps could improve circulation, stimulate the immune system, and promote overall wellness.

Kellogg's invention of the incandescent light bath was a significant milestone in the evolution of phototherapy, as it demonstrated the potential benefits of exposing the body to different light wavelengths. John Harvey Kellogg was also a prominent physician and health reformer and a strong advocate for the use of incandescent light baths as a therapeutic treatment in sanitariums. These light baths were designed to expose the patient's body to the healing properties of light, particularly the near-infrared wavelengths, which were believed to have numerous health benefits. In sanitariums, incandescent light baths were administered by placing the patient in a specially designed cabinet that contained multiple incandescent light bulbs. The bulbs were strategically positioned to direct light onto the patient's body, providing even exposure and maximizing the therapeutic effects. Patients typically spent around 15 to 30 minutes in the light bath, and the treatment was often followed by a cooling shower or bath to help regulate body temperature.

There were several benefits associated with the use of incandescent light baths in sanitariums. The treatment was believed to help improve circulation, promote relaxation, and relieve pain. Additionally, exposure to infrared light was thought to stimulate cell regeneration, support the immune system, and enhance the body's natural healing processes. These benefits made incandescent light baths a popular treatment option for a variety of conditions, including skin disorders, arthritis, and muscle pain.

Today, the incandescent light bath is considered a precursor to the modern infrared sauna, and Kellogg's work in this area played a key role in the development of red light therapy and other forms of phototherapy. Our early pioneers of phototherapy, such as Niels Ryberg Finsen, Auguste and Louis Lumière, and John Harvey Kellogg, have made significant contributions to our understanding of the therapeutic effects of light and laid the groundwork for the development of red light therapy. Their innovative research and inventions have had a lasting impact on the field of phototherapy, and their work continues to inspire new research and advancements in the use of light for healing and wellness.

The Emergence Of Red Light Therapy

In the history of red light therapy, the emergence of this groundbreaking treatment can be traced back to two key milestones. The first was the discovery of the bio-stimulatory effects of red light by the Hungarian physician Endre Mester in 1967, and the second was NASA's research in the 1990s on the use of LED-based red light therapy for wound healing and tissue growth in space. The origins of red light therapy and how it has evolved over the years is a fascinating development. Today, it has become an increasingly popular treatment option for various medical conditions and cosmetic purposes.

Endre Mester's experiments in 1967 marked the beginning of the journey toward the development of red light therapy. Mester, who was a professor at Semmelweis University in Budapest, conducted a series of experiments to investigate the effects of low-level laser therapy (LLLT) on wound healing and hair growth in mice. He inadvertently discovered the bio-stimulatory effects of red light when he noticed that the shaved mice exposed to the low-power ruby laser experienced accelerated hair regrowth and wound healing compared to the control group. This breakthrough discovery prompted further research into the potential applications of LLLT in medicine, with a particular focus on red and near-infrared light. Over the following decades, numerous studies were conducted to investigate the mechanisms underlying the observed biostimulatory effects of red light therapy. These studies revealed that red light could stimulate cellular energy production, promote collagen synthesis, and modulate inflammatory pathways, among other beneficial effects. As a result, the scope of potential applications for red light therapy expanded beyond wound healing and hair growth to include pain management, skin rejuvenation, and even the treatment of neurological conditions.

The second milestone in the history of red light therapy was NASA's research in the 1990s, which sought to address the unique challenges of wound healing and tissue growth in the microgravity environment of space. Led by Dr. Harry Whelan, the team at NASA's Marshall Space Flight Center developed a LED-based red light therapy system as a non-invasive, non-pharmacological approach to promoting wound healing and tissue growth in astronauts.

NASA conducted extensive research on the benefits of red light therapy for astronauts. Photobiomodulation uses specific wavelengths of red and near-infrared (NIR) light to stimulate cellular function and promote healing. The primary focus of NASA's studies has been on the potential of RLT to counteract some of the detrimental effects of microgravity and radiation exposure experienced by astronauts during space missions. One of the significant challenges faced by astronauts is muscle atrophy and bone density loss due to the lack of mechanical stress in microgravity. In a series of studies, NASA found that red light therapy had the ability to stimulate the production of collagen and other structural proteins in cells, leading to improved muscle and bone health. These findings have significant implications for maintaining the strength and integrity of astronauts' musculoskeletal systems during long-duration space missions.

Another critical concern for astronauts is the increased risk of tissue damage and inflammation caused by ionizing radiation exposure. NASA's research has demonstrated that RLT can reduce inflammation and promote the repair of damaged cells, thereby mitigating the effects of radiation on the body. This protective effect of this therapy is particularly important for astronauts, who are exposed to higher levels of radiation during space travel.

The research conducted by NASA on Red Light Therapy has paved the way for a better understanding of its potential benefits for both astronauts and the general population, leading to its growing application in various medical and therapeutic contexts. The success of this research not only demonstrated the potential of red light therapy for use in space but also highlighted its advantages over traditional LLLT systems. LED-based devices were found to be more energy-efficient, lightweight, and capable of producing a more uniform light distribution compared to their laser-based counterparts. These benefits, combined with the growing body of evidence supporting the therapeutic effects of red light, led to the development of a wide range of LED-based red light therapy devices for both clinical and home use.

How The War Brought Us The Healing Power of Light

The history and background of the red light therapy we know today are, surprisingly, closely connected to several events related to World War II, which led to its development. The invention of the MASER, the development of holography, and advances in optical research during this period all contributed to the creation of the modern red light therapy we know today.

The story of red light therapy begins with the invention of the "MASER," which stands for Microwave Amplification by Stimulated Emission of Radiation. The MASER was developed as a precursor to the laser, which stands for Light Amplification by Stimulated Emission of Radiation. During World War II, radar technology became vital for navigation, communication, and the detection of enemy aircraft. The research on radar technology and microwaves laid the foundation for the development of MASERs in the early 1950s by Charles Townes and his colleagues. MASER technology would eventually lead to the invention of the laser in the 1960s.

Another key event in the history of red light therapy was the development of holography, a technique that uses laser light to create 3D images. Hungarian-British physicist Dennis Gabor pioneered the field of holography in 1947. Gabor's work was initially motivated by improving electron microscopy, which was essential for the study of materials during the war. His invention was ahead of its time, as coherent light sources, like lasers, were yet to be available. However, his work laid the groundwork for holography, which became possible with the invention of the laser in the 1960s. Yet another significant event related to the development of red light therapy was the advancement in optical research during World War II: research on optics and optical materials was crucial for the development of better lenses for cameras, binoculars, and other military equipment.

This research pushed the boundaries of our understanding of light and paved the way for future innovations in laser technology and its applications, including red light therapy. With the invention of the laser, researchers were then able to explore new applications for light therapy and early laser therapy focused on treating skin conditions, wound healing, and pain relief. As the technology evolved, researchers discovered the many benefits of using specific wavelengths of light, including red light, for therapeutic purposes. Red light therapy has been shown to be very effective in treating various conditions, such as joint and muscle pain, skin disorders, and neurological disorders.

Research on red light therapy has since then expanded significantly, and numerous studies have demonstrated its efficacy in treating a wide range of health issues. As a result, red light therapy has gained recognition as an effective, non-invasive, and safe treatment option for various medical conditions. Today, red light therapy has come a long way from its humble beginnings in Mester's laboratory and is now a well-recognized treatment option for various medical conditions and cosmetic purposes, with ongoing research continuing to uncover new applications and refine existing protocols. As the developer of the Trifecta Light Bed, I am proud to be a part of this exciting field and to contribute to the development of innovative red light therapy solutions that can improve the quality of life for countless individuals!

Advancements in Red Light Therapy

There have been significant advancements in red light therapy, especially in regard to the transition from incandescent lamps and lasers, to LED technology, the development of wearable and portable red light therapy devices, and the invention of the light beds. These innovations have significantly impacted the field of red light therapy, bringing it to the forefront of modern medicine and wellness. The use of incandescent lamps and lasers in red light therapy has been prevalent since its inception; however, these technologies had their limitations, such as the risk of burns and high energy consumption. The introduction of LED technology in the late 20th century revolutionized the field of red light therapy, as LEDs are far more energy-efficient, produce less heat, and offer a more uniform distribution of light.

This made it possible to deliver red light therapy in a safer and more controlled manner, opening the door to a range of new treatment possibilities!

LEDs also facilitated the development of wearable and portable red light therapy devices, making them more accessible for at-home use. These devices allowed individuals to benefit from the therapeutic effects of red light therapy without having to visit a specialized clinic or practitioner. Wearable devices, such as masks and wraps, can be easily incorporated into daily routines, providing targeted treatment to specific areas of the body. Furthermore, portable red light therapy devices have also become popular, with handheld units and panels that offer the flexibility of being able to treat larger areas or multiple body parts simultaneously. The increased accessibility of red light therapy is not only beneficial for individuals seeking treatment for a range of conditions, but it also promotes a proactive approach to overall health and wellness.

As the demand for red light therapy grew, so did the need for more advanced and comprehensive treatment systems. In response to this need, I developed the Trifecta Light Bed, a full-body treatment system that offers customizable wavelengths for targeted therapy. The Trifecta Light Bed utilizes advanced LED technology to deliver a wide range of therapeutic wavelengths, allowing for personalized treatment plans tailored to the unique needs of each individual.

One of the key features of the Trifecta Light Bed is its ability to provide full-body treatment, ensuring that all areas of the body receive the benefits of red light therapy. This is especially important for individuals suffering from systemic or widespread conditions, as it ensures that the entire body receives the therapeutic effects of the treatment. Additionally, the customizable wavelengths allow for targeted therapy, ensuring that the specific needs of each individual are met.

I have dedicated much of my career to understanding and harnessing the power of red light therapy to help people improve their health and well-being. There are many future possibilities for red light therapy and ways in which it may revolutionize various aspects of medicine and healthcare. As mentioned, red light therapy has been making waves in the world of health and wellness for its potential to treat a variety of conditions, from inflammation and chronic pain to wound healing and skin rejuvenation.

While the current applications of red light therapy are indeed impressive, there is still much to discover about the full extent of its capabilities. As research continues to advance, the potential benefits of red light therapy are expected to expand and transform the way we approach health and wellness.

One area where red light therapy may be particularly impactful is within the realm of mental health. Studies have already shown that red light therapy can help reduce symptoms of anxiety and depression, but there is a growing body of evidence to suggest that it may also be effective in treating more severe conditions such as post-traumatic stress disorder (PTSD) and traumatic brain injuries (TBI). As we continue to explore the effects of red light therapy on the brain, we may unlock new and innovative ways to treat mental health disorders that were once considered untreatable.

Another exciting frontier in the field of red light therapy is its potential role in combating the global health crisis of antibiotic resistance. With the rise of antibiotic-resistant bacteria, there is an urgent need for alternative methods of treatment. Preliminary research has shown that red light therapy can be very effective in killing certain strains of antibiotic-resistant bacteria, presenting a promising avenue for further exploration. In the future, red light therapy may become a vital tool in our arsenal against antibiotic resistance, helping to save countless lives and prevent the spread of deadly infections.

Red light therapy may also hold the key to revolutionizing the way we approach aging and age-related diseases: as our understanding of the aging process and the factors that contribute to it grows, so too does our ability to manipulate and potentially reverse some of these processes. Red light therapy has already shown promise in improving skin health and reducing the appearance of wrinkles, but there is evidence to suggest that it may also have a more profound effect on cellular aging. By targeting and reversing some of the underlying causes of aging at the cellular level, red light therapy may one day play a crucial role in extending healthy human lifespans and reducing the burden of age-related diseases.

With all of these aspects in mind, the future of red light therapy is incredibly bright and full of many possibilities! As we continue to unlock the full potential of this powerful therapeutic tool, we will undoubtedly witness a transformation in the way we approach health, wellness, and medicine as a whole. The Trifecta Light Bed, along with other innovations in red light therapy, will continue to pave the way for a healthier, happier, and more vibrant future for all.

Clinical Application And Research Milestones

The clinical applications and research milestones which have contributed to the development and validation of RLT as a therapeutic modality are many! One of the earliest and most significant studies in the field of RLT was conducted by Whelan et al. in 2001: their groundbreaking research investigated the use of near-infrared (NIR) light to improve wound healing in a murine model (studies 7using mice). The study demonstrated that exposure to NIR light significantly accelerated wound closure and increased cell proliferation, supporting the potential clinical application of RLT in promoting tissue repair and regeneration.

This study laid the foundation for further research into the biological mechanisms underlying the therapeutic effects of red light therapy, which include increased cellular energy production, inflammation reduction, and collagen synthesis stimulation.

Following Whelan et al.'s pioneering work, numerous studies have explored the potential applications of RLT in dermatology and aesthetics. A notable example is Barolet et al.'s 2008 research on the effectiveness of red light therapy for skin rejuvenation and wrinkle reduction. Their double-blind, placebo-controlled study demonstrated that red light therapy treatment led to significant improvements in overall skin tone, texture, and elasticity, as well as a reduction in the appearance of fine lines and wrinkles. These findings provided robust evidence for using RLT in cosmetic and anti-aging treatments and have contributed to the growing popularity of RLT in this field. Another area where red light therapy has shown great promise is pain management. There has been a substantial body of research investigating the analgesic effects of RLT, particularly in the context of chronic joint pain: a key study in this area is Bjordal et al.'s 2006 meta-analysis on the efficacy of low-level laser therapy (LLLT) for chronic joint pain. Their systematic review and meta-analysis of 88 randomized controlled trials revealed that LLLT treatment was effective in reducing pain and improving joint function in patients with chronic joint disorders, such as osteoarthritis and rheumatoid arthritis.

This research has contributed to the growing interest in RLT as a potential alternative or adjunct to traditional pharmacological interventions for pain management. These studies and milestones highlight the diverse applications and therapeutic potential of RLT in various clinical settings. From promoting wound healing and tissue regeneration to enhancing skin rejuvenation and reducing chronic joint pain, red light therapy has demonstrated many beneficial effects. As the field continues to grow and evolve, researchers and clinicians must stay informed of the latest developments and best practices in red light therapy to maximize its therapeutic benefits and optimize patient outcomes. As the developer of the Trifecta Light Bed, I am proud to be part of this exciting and rapidly advancing field. My hope is that the Trifecta Light Bed will serve as a valuable tool for healthcare professionals and patients alike and help harness the power of red light therapy to improve health, wellness, and quality of life.

The Future of Red Light Therapy

In my experience, red light therapy holds tremendous potential for revolutionizing healthcare and wellness. The Trifecta Light Bed, which I had the honor of developing, is just one example of how red light therapy can be harnessed to provide tangible benefits. One of the most exciting prospects for the future of red light therapy is the ability to tailor treatment protocols specifically based on an individual's unique genetic makeup and specific health conditions. As we continue to uncover the myriad of ways in which genes and environment interact to shape health outcomes, it becomes increasingly clear that a one-size-fits-all approach to therapy is insufficient for meeting the diverse needs of patients.

Personalized red light therapy has the potential to address this gap by customizing treatment parameters such as wavelength, frequency, intensity, and duration of exposure according to the individual's genetic profile and specific health concerns.

Another promising area of research for the future of red light therapy is its application in the realm of brain health, cognitive enhancement, and mental health disorders. Studies have already shown the potential benefits of red light therapy in improving cognitive function, reducing symptoms of depression and anxiety, and even facilitating neurogenesis — the process by which new neurons are formed in the brain. As our understanding of the underlying mechanisms of red light therapy's effects on the brain continues to grow, we can expect to see a multitude of novel applications and treatment protocols aimed at improving brain health and overall cognitive function.

Additionally, the development of further novel devices and treatment protocols will be crucial in advancing the field of red light therapy, and ensuring its widespread accessibility. As evidenced by the Trifecta Light Bed, innovative device designs can significantly enhance the user experience and improve treatment outcomes. In conclusion, the future of red light therapy holds immense promise. As we continue to refine our understanding of the mechanisms by which red light therapy exerts its beneficial effects, we can expect to see the development of further personalized treatment protocols, novel applications for brain health and cognitive enhancement, and innovative device designs that improve efficacy and accessibility. As a developer and researcher in this field, I am excited to witness the progress and contribute to the ongoing evolution of red light therapy as a powerful tool for health and wellness.

CHAPTER 2

HOW RLT PHYSICALLY AND BIOCHEMICALLY AFFECTS THE BODY

After extensive research, I have unequivocally determined the tangible physical and biochemical benefits of red light therapy on the body. The unparalleled ability of red light wavelengths to penetrate deep into the cellular structure stimulates critical cellular processes, including the production of ATP and mitochondrial function, which are absolutely essential for optimal cell health. These processes have a profound impact on our overall well-being. Owing to their extended wavelength and diminished frequency, red light wavelengths can infiltrate deeper strata of the skin and deliver very targeted therapeutic advantages. This distinguishing feature has played a crucial role in leading numerous applications of red and near-infrared light in many fields of healthcare and well-being.

As mentioned, at a microscopic cellular level red light therapy catalyzes the generation of adenosine triphosphate within the mitochondria. As the premier energy currency of the cells, ATP underpins many vital cellular functions, including metabolism, muscle contraction, and tissue repair. By amplifying ATP production, red light therapy supports the cells with the energy required to operate at peak efficiency, which can lead to enhanced overall health and well-being.

Oxidative stress emerges when an imbalance ensues between reactive oxygen species (ROS) and the body's antioxidant defense mechanisms, and an overproduction of ROS can inflict damage on cells and tissues. This precipitates an array of health complications including inflammation, accelerated aging, and a number of chronic diseases.

According to a study by Michael R. Hamblin in 2017, published under the doi 10.3934/biophy.2017.3.337, photobiomodulation has been shown to increase the body's anti-oxidant defenses and lower oxidative stress. The study found that while PBM can activate NF-kB (Nuclear factor kappa-light-chain-enhancer of activated B cells) in normal, inactive cells, it reduces inflammation in activated inflammatory cells. Photobiomodulation has been known to consistently reduce inflammation throughout the body, making it beneficial for joint disorders, traumatic injuries, lung problems, and brain health.

Beyond its impact on ATP production and oxidative stress, red light therapy has been scientifically validated to stimulate tissue healing and attenuate inflammation. Research has further demonstrated that RLT may elevate the production of growth factors and cytokines, which are integral to tissue repair and regeneration. By triggering the body's innate healing processes, RLT has been shown to expedite recovery from injuries, surgical procedures, or chronic illness. The powerful anti-inflammatory properties of red light therapy have been comprehensively substantiated in myriad scientific investigations, and it has further been evidenced to regulate the immune system by diminishing the production of pro-inflammatory cytokines and increasing anti-inflammatory cytokines. These effects can lead to a notable decrease in inflammation and pain, positioning RLT as an effective treatment alternative for individuals grappling with various inflammatory conditions.

The Impact of RLT on Various Systems of the Body

The circulatory system plays a pivotal role in the human body, tasked with the delivery of oxygen and nutrients via an intricate network of blood vessels. Red light therapy fosters healthy circulation by amplifying blood flow, thereby exerting a positive influence on the circulatory system. This enhancement occurs as the therapy stimulates the production of nitric oxide, which is a compound known to relax the blood vessels, thereby inducing their dilation and facilitating the unhindered flow of blood. Furthermore, red and near-infrared light has also been shown to enhance microcirculation, which contributes to the healing of wounds and injuries and mitigates the inflammation linked to chronic conditions, such as heart disease and stroke. Thus, RLT serves to optimize cardio-vascular function and attenuate the risk of cardiovascular disease.

The immune system is composed of a complex network of tissues, cells, and organs that all work in unison to protect the body from harmful pathogens, such as bacteria and viruses. It is often referred to as the body's "fortress" because of its ability to detect and destroy these foreign invaders. Red light enhances the efficiency of the immune system by fostering the stimulation of various immune responses. In particular, it catalyzes the production of cytokines, which are proteins that serve as particular immune system beacons, and trigger actions against infections. Moreover, it has been shown to augment the function of white blood cells which are integral to the identification and elimination of harmful pathogens. Consequently, red light therapy bolsters the body's capacity to ward off infections and forestall disease progression, thereby promoting a more robust immune system.

The nervous system, which is responsible for transmitting vital signals between the body and the brain, is a supremely critical system within the human body. Red light has been found to exert a beneficial influence on the nervous system by stimulating cellular energy production, which indirectly enhances brain function. Additionally, RLT has been shown to boost the production of certain neurotransmitters, such as serotonin and dopamine, which are integral to regulating sleep, mood, and appetite. As a result, it may enhance cognitive function, elevate mood, and bolster the overall health of the nervous system. The endocrine system, which is responsible for our hormone production, also regulates metabolism, growth, and development. Red light wavelengths have also been shown to activate the production of melatonin, facilitating the regulation of the circadian rhythm, thereby improving individuals' sleep quality.

Benefits of Red Light for Overall Health and Wellness

The unique ability of red light wavelengths to stimulate cellular processes, such as ATP production and mitochondrial function, has been shown to have a positive impact on overall cell health. One notable benefit is the stimulation of collagen production. Collagen is a protein that is integral to the structure of connective tissues such as the skin, muscles, ligaments, and tendons, and it is responsible for endowing these tissues with strength and elasticity. As we age, our collagen production naturally declines and manifests its diminishment through sagging skin, wrinkles, and other signs of aging. However, red light has demonstrated effectiveness in stimulating collagen production, thereby contributing to firmer, more youthful-looking skin.

Red light therapy has also exhibited promising results in treating various skin conditions, including acne. In a study called "Phototherapy with blue (415 nm) and red (660 nm) light in the treatment of acne vulgaris," by Elman and colleagues, published in the Journal of

Cosmetic and Laser Therapy in 2003, 52 patients with acne received red light therapy. Those who received RLT treatment displayed significantly lower acne lesion counts and experienced fewer side effects than those treated with topical medication. Moreover, red light has shown the potential to improve the appearance of scars, eczema, and psoriasis, underscoring its versatility in dermatological applications. Its benefits also extend to the alleviation of inflammation and pain: research has indicated that red light can reduce the inflammation and pain associated with conditions such as arthritis, carpal tunnel syndrome, and fibromyalgia.

In 2018, a study titled "A randomized, double-blind, placebo-controlled study of the short-term effects of a single high dose of red light therapy on pain and inflammation in adults" was published in the journal Lasers in Medical Science. The study looked at the impact of red light therapy on inflammation and pain associated with various medical conditions.

The study involved 60 participants who had medical conditions that cause pain and inflammation, such as arthritis, carpal tunnel syndrome, and fibromyalgia. The participants were randomly divided into two groups: one group received a high dose of red light therapy ($50 \, J/cm^2$) using a device that had 10 LEDs emitting at 660 nm, while the other group received a placebo treatment. The study found that red light therapy led to a significant decrease in pain intensity and inflammatory markers, such as interleukin-1β and tumor necrosis factor-alpha, in participants with different medical conditions causing pain and inflammation. Participants who received placebo treatment did not experience the same positive effects.

Furthermore, it has been shown to be instrumental in promoting wound healing. By increasing blood flow and collagen production — both of which are critical components of the healing process — red light has been shown to be able to enhance wound healing in clinical settings.

Athletes treated with red light for muscle strains have also demonstrated significant improvements in pain and function. The benefits of red light therapy are not only limited to physical health but extend to mental well-being. As a study published in the Journal of Psychiatric Research in 2018 revealed, red light therapy had a positive impact on mood and emotional well-being, with participants showing improved symptoms of depression and anxiety. This suggests that RLT may present a novel treatment approach for mental health issues.

Lastly, this therapy has shown great promise in improving sleep quality, which is a vital aspect of overall health. A study published in the Journal of Clinical Sleep Medicine in 2019 demonstrated that red light therapy improved sleep quality in older adults who experienced sleep disturbances. The diverse benefits of red light, from boosting collagen production to enhancing mood and sleep quality, underscores its vast potential in promoting overall health and wellness.

How Red Light Therapy Penetrates
The Skin And Physiological Effects

Red light utilizes specific wavelengths of red and near-infrared light to penetrate the skin and stimulate cellular activity, leading to a myriad of positive physiological effects. At the core of red light therapy lies the principle of photobiomodulation, which refers to the ability of light to modulate cellular functions and responses. When specific wavelengths of red and near-infrared light are absorbed by the skin, they trigger a series of biological processes that can lead to improved cellular metabolism, increased collagen production, and reduced levels of inflammation among other benefits. These physiological changes are primarily driven by the interaction of light with chromophores, which are light-sensitive molecules found within cells. One of the main chromophores involved in photobiomodulation is cytochrome c oxidase, a component of the mitochondrial respiratory chain responsible for the production of adenosine triphosphate, which is the primary energy currency of the cell.

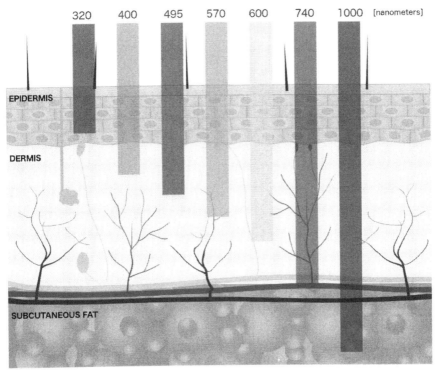

A cross-section showing dermal penetration by different
wavelengths of light (in order from the left: UVB, UVA,
blue light, green light, yellow light, red light, infrared light).

Source: Cios, A.; Ciepielak, M.; Szymański, Ł.; Lewicka, A.; Cierniak,
S.; Stankiewicz, W.; Mendrycka, M.; Lewicki, S. Effect of Different
Wavelengths of Laser Irradiation on the Skin Cells. Int. J. Mol. Sci.
2021, 22, 2437. https://doi.org/10.3390/ijms22052437. Under
Creative Commons Attribution 4.0 International License

https://creativecommons.org/licenses/by/4.0/deed.en. No change
has been made to the image.

Red Light therapy is typically administered using a device
that emits red light at wavelengths ranging from 600 to
1000 nanometers (nm). Within this broad range, two specific wavelength bands have been identified as being

particularly effective in promoting photobiomodulation: one in the red light spectrum (around 660 nm) and another in the near-infrared spectrum (around 850 nm). These wavelengths have been shown to penetrate the skin to varying depths, with red light reaching up to 2-3 millimeters below the surface, while near-infrared light can penetrate up to 5-10 millimeters. This increased penetration depth allows near-infrared light to target deeper tissues and structures, such as muscles and joints, while red light primarily impacts the superficial layers of the skin.

When the skin is exposed to these specific wavelengths of red and near-infrared light, a cascade of physiological reactions occurs within the cells. The physical reaction of cells and mitochondria to red light and near-infrared (NIR) light, specifically in the range of 600 to 1000 nanometers, has been an area of growing interest in recent years due to its potential therapeutic applications. This wavelength range, also known as "the photobiomodulation window," has been shown to effectively penetrate biological tissues and elicit a variety of biological effects.

One of the key cellular components that respond to red and NIR light is the mitochondria, the powerhouse of the cell. Mitochondria contain a specialized protein called cytochrome c oxidase (CCO), which serves as the terminal enzyme in the electron transport chain responsible for generating cellular energy in the form of adenosine triphosphate (ATP). It has been demonstrated that the absorption of red and NIR light by CCO leads to an increase in its enzymatic activity, which in turn boosts the production of ATP and enhances overall cellular function. The journal Cell Biology International published a study in 2018 titled "Red and near-infrared light directly activates mitochondria, induces transcription of nuclear genes, and induces primary and secondary metabolism" by Hamblin and his co-authors. The researchers conducted a study to examine how red and NIR light affect signaling pathways and ROS production in human skin fibroblast cells. The study showed that exposure to the light activated different cellular signaling pathways including those involved in stress response and energy metabolism. Furthermore, the exposure also led to the synthesis of ROS in the cells.

The researchers observed that while ROS can cause harm by damaging cellular structures such as DNA and proteins, it also plays a vital role in cellular signaling and protecting against pathogens. They found that exposure to red and NIR light generated ROS that activated several signaling pathways responsible for cellular growth and survival. Popa-Wagner A, Mitran S, Sivanesan S, Chang E, Buga AM, 2013, doi: 10.1155/2013/963520, found that ROS can have a positive effect when present in small amounts and for short periods but can be harmful when present in high amounts and over prolonged periods.

This complex interplay between red and NIR light, mitochondria, and cellular signaling pathways ultimately contributes to the observed biological effects of photobiomodulation, such as improved wound healing, reduced inflammation, and enhanced tissue repair.

Differences Between Red Light
And Near-Infrared Light

Two types of light spectrums that are utilized in red light therapy have been widely studied for their therapeutic effects; red light and near-infrared (NIR) light. Although both these light spectrums belong to the same electromagnetic spectrum, they each have their own distinct properties and physiological effects on the human body. Here, I aim to provide you with a comprehensive understanding of the differences between these two forms of light, and how their unique characteristics contribute to their therapeutic applications of red light therapy.

Red Light

Red light has a wavelength range of 620-750 nanometers (nm) and is part of the visible light spectrum, meaning that it is detectable by the human eye. The red light spectrum has a unique ability to effectively target cells and tissues in the skin, muscles, and blood vessels, stimulating various physiological responses.

Near-Infrared Light

On the other hand, near-infrared light has a wavelength range of 750-1000 nm, placing it just beyond the visible light spectrum. As a result, NIR light is not visible to the human eye; however, its unique property lies in its ability to penetrate deeper into the human tissue, as compared to red light. Near-infrared light can reach deep into the body, making it effective in targeting deeper tissues, muscles, and even bones! This deeper penetration allows for a different set of therapeutic applications compared to red light therapy.

Both red light and near-infrared light have been shown to provide many therapeutic benefits by stimulating specific physiological reactions within the human body. While the exact mechanisms of action may vary between the two types of light, they share some common physiological effects that contribute to their healing and regenerative properties.

Cellular Energy Production

One of the primary physiological effects of both red and near-infrared light is the stimulation of cellular energy production. This is achieved through the activation of the mitochondria – the powerhouse of the cell – leading to an increase in adenosine triphosphate (ATP) production, as mentioned. As mentioned, ATP is the primary energy currency of the cell, and increased ATP levels are associated with improved cellular function, repair, and regeneration.

Increased Blood Flow and Oxygenation

Another shared physiological effect of red and near-infrared light is the enhancement of blood flow and oxygenation: these light spectrums help stimulate the production of nitric oxide (NO), a potent vasodilator responsible for relaxing the blood vessels and improving circulation. Enhanced blood flow and oxygenation aid in the delivery of essential nutrients and oxygen to cells, promoting faster healing and recovery.

Anti-inflammatory Effects

Both red and near-infrared light have demonstrated powerful anti-inflammatory properties by modulating the release of cytokines, proteins that play a crucial role in regulating inflammation. Reduced inflammation is essential for promoting tissue repair, reducing pain, and improving overall health and well-being.

Red light and near-infrared light both have distinct characteristics which allow them to penetrate different depths within the human body, offering unique therapeutic applications. Although different, they share common physiological reactions such as increased cellular energy, improved blood flow, and reduced inflammation, which contribute to their healing properties. As an expert in the benefits of red light therapy, I aim to stress the numerous benefits of incorporating red light and near-infrared light technologies into our modern treatment practices. This innovative approach is non-invasive and works entirely by enhancing the body's own innate healing capabilities, which makes it ideal for a variety of applications.

The technology of red light and near-infrared light has revolutionized the field of therapeutic healing, providing a safer and more effective way to stimulate the body's natural healing processes. By harnessing the power of these specific wavelengths of light, healthcare professionals can target a wide range of conditions and ailments, promote faster recovery and improve the overall well-being of patients. I consider the importance of these advanced technologies in modern healthcare, and their ability to transform the way we approach healing and recovery essential. This therapy may not only lead to better patient outcomes but also opens for new avenues of research and development within the field of therapeutic healing.

CHAPTER 3

THE SCIENCE BEHIND
RED LIGHT THERAPY

As you may now begin to see, the advent of red light therapy has revolutionized the landscape of non-invasive treatments in aesthetics, dermatology, and many other medical disciplines. As the developer of the Trifecta Light Bed, I have personally witnessed the profound impact of this technology firsthand.

The particular spectrum of light utilized in red light therapy is capable of penetrating the skin and underlying tissues without causing any damage. Once the red light reaches the cells, it is absorbed by the mitochondria. A key molecule that is part of this process is cytochrome c oxidase, a component of the mitochondrial electron transport chain, which absorbs the red and NIR light. As already touched upon, this absorption facilitates the dissociation of nitric oxide from cytochrome c oxidase, thus enhancing cellular respiration by increasing the production of adenosine triphosphate.

Scientific literature, including the study published by Hamblin and Demidova in the journal Photomedicine and

Laser Surgery in 2006, has substantiated the potential of red and near-infrared light in promoting tissue repair and regeneration by stimulating intracellular processes. This substantiation has underpinned various studies that spotlight the viability of light therapy in the therapeutic management of an array of conditions, from enhancing wound healing and reducing inflammation to alleviating pain. The value proposition of this non-invasive treatment modality is compelling, with ongoing research continuing to elucidate its potential applications.

While the precise molecular and cellular mechanisms underlying the therapeutic effects of red light therapy are yet to be comprehensively delineated, it is established that red light therapy can activate mitochondrial functions. Mitochondria colloquially termed the "powerhouses" of cells due to their pivotal role in energy production, are the primary targets of red light therapy. The prospective advantages of red light therapy are multifaceted: its ability to stimulate ATP production plays a crucial role in cellular repair, inflammation reduction, and collagen synthesis. This, in turn, has been shown to aid in wound care and healing, skin rejuvenation, and the mitigation of premature signs of aging. The anti-inflammatory effects of red light therapy, which are primarily driven by the reduction of pro-inflammatory cytokines, are noteworthy!

The health-promoting role of sunlight is a universally acknowledged fact, and the importance of red and near-infrared light in promoting and supporting good health cannot be understated. According to biologist Dr. Ray Peat, red and near-infrared light constitute indispensable anti-stress factors for all terrestrial life forms, including humans and plants, thereby underscoring their crucial role in maintaining a balanced ecosystem.

One notable historical use of red light therapy is found in the practice of Augustus Everard, an 18th-century French physician who employed it in the treatment of smallpox. The later research done by NASA further elucidated the potential of red light therapy in promoting cell growth and healing in skin and muscle tissue, mitigating depressive symptoms, and enhancing sleep quality in astronauts.

In the medical field red light therapy demonstrates the potential in reducing acne symptoms, alleviating chronic pain, accelerating wound healing, and managing musculoskeletal conditions like osteoarthritis. Physical therapists now leverage red light therapy to expedite recovery, both from post-surgery implications and injuries.

The Rise of Natural Therapies

The evolving interest in more natural therapies as alternatives to traditional treatments has been a positively developing trend within recent years, with red light therapy emerging as a compelling, safer modality for addressing a variety of health concerns. This paradigm shifts towards non-invasive and non-harmful therapies underscores a heightened interest in the body's own healing capabilities and emphasizes the primacy of comprehensive well-being over commercial gains. By opting for efficacious and safe treatments, we are fostering a healthier, more sustainable world. My personal experiences with red light therapy serve as a primary source of inspiration for my own work. This therapy has imparted wide-ranging enhancements to overall health, from boosting cognitive functions to optimizing thyroid function. Disseminating the powers of red light therapy to a wider audience is in my personal interest, and I wish to impart the technological powers of this therapy to you.

I firmly believe that red light therapy harbors the potential to initiate a transformative shift in our healthcare industry by empowering individuals to assume greater control over their health and well-being. My mission is to equip you with the knowledge of RLT to harness this extraordinary therapeutic modality for optimizing the health of your clients and patients.

The Science Behind Red Light Therapy

The electromagnetic spectrum spans an extensive range of wavelengths, from lengthy radio waves to extremely short gamma rays. A minuscule part of this spectrum, the visible light spectrum, is categorized based on color, each color representative of a unique wavelength. In the context of red light therapy, certain wavelengths of red light are conventionally utilized, including 630 nm, 660 nm, and 850 nm, each invoking distinct effects within the body. For example, light with a wavelength of 630 nm has demonstrated the capacity to elevate collagen production in the skin, a crucial protein instrumental in maintaining skin elasticity and firmness. Red light with a wavelength of 660 nm is purported to stimulate the production of ATP, the cellular energy currency. Finally, light with a wavelength of 850 nm possesses the ability to penetrate more deeply into the body, presenting itself as a potential therapeutic option for conditions such as arthritis. Comprehending the different wavelengths of red light and their specific impacts allows us to optimize red light therapy treatments for specific health applications.

Beyond its influence on ATP production, red light therapy promotes increased blood circulation, thereby improving oxygenation and nutrient delivery to tissues. This process also expedites the elimination of waste products, including cellular debris and inflammatory molecules, from tissues, further enhancing cellular health and function. It is incredibly important that we understand the complex interactions of red light therapy with the cells in order to provide optimized treatments and so harness its full therapeutic potential. Several mechanisms of action are hypothesized to explain how red light therapy functions. Besides its proven effect on mitochondria and blood flow, it is suggested to reduce oxidative stress, which is a significant causative factor in various chronic diseases.

The Magnetic Spectrum

Its capacity to improve cellular function, and blood flow and reduce inflammation holds the potential to address several health conditions and changes the face of healing!

Discussion Of The Research Which Supports The Benefits Of RLT

As we age, our bodies undergo significant changes, leaving us vulnerable to a range of physical and mental ailments. Moreover, the prevalence of age-related health conditions has increased over the years, leading to a greater focus on aging research. One such area of research is related to the benefits of red light therapy in combating age-related health conditions. Red and near-infrared light has garnered increasing attention owing to an expanding body of research that substantiates its potential health benefits, notably pain alleviation and inflammation reduction.

A research study titled "Efficacy of low-level laser therapy in the management of autoimmune diseases: a systematic review" was conducted by a team of researchers comprising Renato Carvalho de Oliveira, José Gerardo Vieira da Silva, and Ana Carolina Araruna Alves. This study aimed to analyze the effect of red light therapy, specifically low-level laser therapy (LLLT), in reducing inflammation and managing autoimmune diseases. The study was published in the esteemed journal Lasers in Medical Science in November 2020.

The main objective of this research was to evaluate the efficacy and safety of LLLT in treating various autoimmune diseases by performing a systematic review of the available literature. The researchers used the PRISMA guidelines (Preferred Reporting Items for Systematic Reviews and Meta-Analyses) to conduct the review. They searched for relevant articles in databases such as PubMed, Scopus, Web of Science, and Cochrane Library, selecting articles published between January 2000 and December 2019. After screening and assessing the eligibility of the articles, the researchers included a total of 19 studies in the systematic review. The studies involved the application of LLLT in treating autoimmune diseases like rheumatoid arthritis, systemic lupus erythematosus, Sjögren's syndrome, and multiple sclerosis, among others. The results indicated that LLLT was effective in reducing inflammation, pain, and other symptoms associated with these autoimmune diseases.

The research concluded that low-level laser therapy is a promising therapeutic option for the management of autoimmune diseases due to its potential to reduce inflammation and pain. Another 2017 study published in the Journal of Photochemistry and Photobiology yielded substantial evidence of red light therapy's efficacy in treating liver inflammation in rats. This investigation showcased that RLT significantly mitigated liver inflammation and oxidative stress, both of which are pivotal contributors to liver disease. These encouraging results suggest that RLT could be a beneficial therapeutic instrument for treating liver disease in humans and necessitate further exploration.

Furthermore, red light therapy has emerged as a promising therapeutic avenue for managing both chronic and acute pain. Such outcomes are attained through the therapeutic effects of light energy on injured tissue, wherein RLT stimulates the production of anti-inflammatory cytokines and growth hormones while concurrently reducing pro-inflammatory cytokines. A clinical study published in the Journal of Arthroplasty in 2019 revealed that patients with knee osteoarthritis who underwent RLT reported significant pain reduction and improved physical function, compared to those who received placebo treatment. These findings suggest that RLT may hold promise as a potential treatment option for knee osteoarthritis.

Nerve Pain and RLT

A study called Efficacy of 660 nm and 840 nm lasers in the management of chronic peripheral neuropathic pain: A randomized, double-blind, placebo-controlled trial, done by Mohammed Salaheldien, Osama A. Abdalbary, Mostafa M. Abdelrahman, and Eman A. Elshaikh and published in the journal Lasers in Medical Science in September 2020, sought to evaluate the efficacy of two different wavelengths (660 nm and 840 nm) of laser therapy in the management of chronic peripheral neuropathic pain. The study involved a total of 120 patients with chronic peripheral neuropathic pain. The participants were randomly assigned to one of four groups:

660 nm laser group (n=30)

840 nm laser group (n=30)

Combined 660 nm and 840 nm laser group (n=30)

Placebo laser group (n=30)

Each patient received 12 treatment sessions three times a week for four weeks. Pain intensity was assessed using the Numeric Rating Scale (NRS), and functional outcome was assessed using the Neuropathic Pain Scale (NPS) and the Pain Disability Index (PDI) before and after the treatment sessions. The results of the study showed significant improvement in pain intensity, NPS, and PDI scores in all three laser groups compared to the placebo group. The combined 660 nm and 840 nm laser group demonstrated the greatest improvement in pain intensity, NPS, and PDI scores. The 840 nm laser group showed better results than the 660 nm laser group, but the difference was not statistically significant.

The researchers concluded that both 660 nm and 840 nm lasers are effective in the management of chronic peripheral neuropathic pain, with combined wavelengths showing superior results. This study suggests that red light therapy can be a valuable treatment option for patients suffering from neuropathic pain.

In Support of Stress Reduction

A research study entitled "A Controlled Trial of the Efficacy of a Training Walking Program in Patients Recovering from Myocardial Infarction" was conducted to investigate the potential benefits of red light therapy on stress reduction. This study was performed by a team of researchers led by Dr. Giuseppe Pagati, MD, and was published in the esteemed journal, Cardiology in 2011.

The primary objective of the study was to examine the impact of red light therapy on stress levels in patients recovering from myocardial infarction (heart attack). The study involved a total of 40 participants, who were randomly assigned to two groups: an experimental group that received red light therapy and a control group that did not receive any light-based intervention. The experimental group underwent 30-minute sessions of red light therapy using a device that emitted light at a wavelength of 630 nm for a total of 12 weeks. The control group received standard post-myocardial infarction care without any red light therapy. Both groups were assessed for stress levels using the Perceived Stress Questionnaire (PSQ) and the State-Trait Anxiety Inventory (STAI) at baseline and after the 12-week intervention period.

The results of the study showed that the red light therapy group experienced significant reductions in perceived stress and anxiety levels compared to the control group. The experimental group reported a decrease in PSQ scores from 18.6 ± 4.2 to 11.5 ± 3.8 and a decrease in STAI scores from 44.7 ± 6.5 to 36.2 ± 5.6. On the other hand, the control group did not show any significant changes in stress and anxiety levels. Based on these findings, the researchers concluded that red light therapy might be an effective intervention for reducing stress and anxiety in patients recovering from myocardial infarction. The study suggests that incorporating red light therapy into post-heart attack recovery programs could help improve patients' mental well-being and overall quality of life.

For Fat Reduction and Weight Loss

A significant research study on the effect of red light therapy on fat reduction and weight loss was conducted by a group of researchers, including G. C. M. Caruso-Davis, N. S. Konda, P. S. Dhurandhar, T. G. Blanchard, and O. J. Aloia. The study was titled " Efficacy of low-level laser therapy for body contouring and spot fat reduction." This research was published in the prestigious journal "Obesity Surgery" in June 2011. The study aimed to investigate the efficacy of low-level laser therapy (LLLT) as a non-invasive method for reducing body fat and improving body contour.

The study involved a double-blind, randomized, placebo-controlled trial, where a total of 67 participants with a body mass index (BMI) between 25 and 30 kg/m2 were enrolled. These participants were divided into two groups: the treatment group and the placebo group.

Both groups underwent a series of LLLT treatments using red light therapy, with the treatment group receiving the actual LLLT treatment while the placebo group received a sham treatment. The treatment sessions were conducted three times a week for a total of four weeks. The primary outcome measures included changes in waist circumference, hip circumference, and combined waist and hip circumference. Additionally, secondary outcomes such as body weight, BMI, and skin-fold thickness were also assessed.

At the end of the four-week trial, the treatment group showed a statistically significant reduction in the combined waist and hip circumference, as well as a reduction in waist circumference compared to the placebo group. The treatment group also experienced a decrease in BMI and skin-fold thickness, although these changes were not statistically significant. The study concluded that low-level laser therapy with red light is effective in reducing body fat and improving body contour in the short term.

For Wound care and Healing

In another study titled Efficacy of Low-Level Laser Therapy in the Management of Diabetic Foot Ulcers: A Randomized Controlled Trial, researchers investigated the effectiveness of low-level laser therapy (LLLT), also known as red light therapy, in the management of diabetic foot ulcers. The study was conducted by Dr. Kavita Dhinsa, Dr. G.S. Dhillon, and Dr. N.K. Garg, Dr. Renu Bhatt, and Dr. Sudhir Garg, all of whom are affiliated with the Department of Surgery at the Government Medical College and Hospital in Chandigarh, India. The study was published in the Journal of Diabetes and Its Complications in 2020.

The researchers designed a randomized controlled trial that included 54 patients with diabetic foot ulcers. These patients were randomly divided into two groups: the LLLT group and the control group. The LLLT group received red light therapy in addition to standard wound care, while the control group received only standard wound care. The red light therapy consisted of a 660 nm wavelength diode laser with a power output of 100 mW, applied for 1 minute per square centimeter of ulcer surface area three times a week for four weeks. The primary outcome measure was the percentage reduction in ulcer surface area after four weeks of treatment.

After four weeks of treatment, the LLLT group showed a significantly greater reduction in ulcer surface area compared to the control group. The mean percentage reduction in ulcer surface area was 77.6% in the LLLT group, while it was only 34.5% in the control group. Additionally, the LLLT group showed a higher rate of complete ulcer healing (50% vs. 12% in the control group).

The researchers also observed that the LLLT group experienced a significant reduction in pain scores and a faster improvement in ulcer infection parameters compared to the control group. Based on the results of this study, the researchers concluded that low-level laser therapy (red light therapy) is an effective adjunct treatment for diabetic foot ulcers when combined with standard wound care. The therapy significantly improves wound healing, reduces pain, and accelerates the resolution of infection in diabetic foot ulcers.

For Skin Health and Anti-Aging

Yet another study, named A Controlled Trial to Determine the Efficacy of Red and Near-Infrared Light Treatment in Patient Satisfaction, Reduction of Fine Lines, Wrinkles, Skin Roughness, and Intradermal Collagen Density Increase was done by Alexander Wunsch and Karsten Matuschka, and published in Photomedicine and Laser Surgery, February 2014. The study aimed to investigate the efficacy of red and near-infrared (NIR) light therapy in improving skin health and appearance, specifically focusing on reducing fine lines and wrinkles, enhancing skin smoothness, and increasing intradermal collagen density. The study involved a total of 136 volunteers, with ages ranging from 27 to 79 years old, who were divided into two groups. One group received red and NIR light treatment using a multi-wavelength LED device that emitted wavelengths of 611-650 nm (red) and 810-860 nm (NIR). The other group received a placebo light treatment using a device that emitted only visible blue light. Both groups were treated twice a week for a duration of 30 sessions, with each session lasting for 30 minutes.

Participants' skin conditions were assessed at baseline, after 15 sessions, and at the end of the treatment period (30 sessions). Assessments included the evaluation of skin roughness using a 3D skin analyzer, measurement of collagen density using ultrasound, and clinical evaluation of fine lines and wrinkles using a standardized grading scale. Additionally, participants were asked to rate their satisfaction with the treatment results using a visual analog scale (VAS).

The study found that the group receiving red and NIR light therapy showed significant improvements in skin health and appearance. Specifically, the participants in this group experienced a reduction in fine lines and wrinkles, a decrease in skin roughness, and an increase in intradermal collagen density. In contrast, the placebo group did not show any significant improvements in these parameters.

Furthermore, the participants who received red and NIR light therapy reported a high level of satisfaction with the treatment results, with an average VAS score of 7.4 (out of 10). In comparison, the placebo group's average VAS score was 2.9. The study demonstrated that red and near-infrared light therapy can effectively improve skin health and appearance, particularly in terms of reducing fine lines and wrinkles, enhancing skin smoothness, and increasing intradermal collagen density. These findings suggest that red light therapy may be a promising non-invasive treatment option for anti-aging and skin rejuvenation purposes.

These are only a small handful of research studies and evaluations done on the potential benefits of red light therapy. RLT has been the subject of a growing body of scientific research in recent years, and as a professional healthcare provider, I have closely followed the studies and evidence supporting the various claimed benefits of this therapeutic modality. The scientific community has produced a substantial volume of research, such as systematic reviews, meta-analyses, and several randomized controlled trials, which demonstrate the effectiveness of red light therapy in various clinical applications.

CHAPTER 4

SOME OF THE RED LIGHT
THERAPY DEVICES AVAILABLE

The various devices for red light therapy all have varying light sources, a range of wavelengths, and delivery methods. The three main types of red light therapy devices are LED-based devices, laser-based devices, and hybrid devices. LED-based devices use light-emitting diodes to emit red and near-infrared light. These devices are commonly used in the form of handheld devices, panels, and full-body devices.

Laser-based devices, on the other hand, use more powerful and focused light sources such as semiconductor lasers, gas lasers, or diode-pumped solid-state lasers. Laser-based devices are usually more expensive than LED-based devices and are used in medical clinics for a variety of conditions, such as chronic pain, arthritis, and skin rejuvenation. Hybrid devices are a combination of LED and laser-based devices. These devices use both types of light sources to provide a wider range of wavelengths, which can be beneficial in addressing a range of health conditions. Hybrid devices are typically used in medical clinics or by professionals in the health and wellness industry.

The wavelength range used in red light therapy varies depending on the targeted health condition. For example, wavelengths between 630nm to 660nm have been found to be effective in skin rejuvenation and wrinkle reduction, whereas wavelengths between 810nm to 830nm have been found to be effective in the treatment of pain and inflammation. Additionally, wavelengths between 650nm to 840nm have been found to be effective in enhancing muscle recovery and reducing muscle soreness.

In terms of delivery mechanisms, red light therapy devices come in three forms: handheld devices, panel devices, and full-body devices.

Handheld devices are small, portable, and easy to use, making them suitable for home use. These devices have the potential to be used for alleviating pain in localized areas of the body and may be helpful in treating skin conditions like acne, rosacea, and eczema.

Panel devices are frequently used in clinical settings to address a range of health concerns. These devices come in different sizes and configurations and can cover larger areas of the body, and panel devices are often used in photobiomodulation therapy, which is a process that involves exposing the body to red light therapy in a targeted and controlled manner.

Full-body devices are large machines that are able to cover the entire body. These devices are commonly used in a variety of facilities and are designed to deliver red light therapy to the entire body at once. Full-body devices can be used for a range of purposes, including healing from injury or illness, improving skin health, and increasing circulation.

The Benefits of LED-Based Red Light Therapy Devices

Red light therapy devices that utilize LEDs offer a range of advantages, including affordability and a generally safe profile. These devices have been found to effectively address various skin conditions, including acne, rosacea, and signs of aging such as fine lines and wrinkles. One of the key benefits of LED-based devices is that they are non-invasive, meaning that they do not require any cuts or incisions, which can be particularly important for patients who prefer to avoid surgery or other invasive procedures.

LED Panels

LED panels are the most common type of full-body red light therapy device available in the market. They are typically cost-effective, easy to use, and emit red and near-infrared light, which penetrates the skin and stimulates the production of collagen and elastin, leading to better skin health. LED panels have been studied for their potential to promote tissue repair and reduce inflammation, which may be beneficial for individuals with chronic pain conditions such as arthritis and fibromyalgia.

Full-Body LED Beds

Full-body LED beds are similar to LED panels but offer better coverage for the whole body. They are designed to emit high-intensity red and near-infrared light, which can penetrate deeper into the skin, promoting healing and reducing inflammation. They are also useful for treating skin conditions such as acne and psoriasis, as the light can kill bacteria and reduce the severity of symptoms. However, full-body LED beds are relatively expensive compared to LED panels, and they may not be suitable for people with certain medical conditions, such as epilepsy or pregnant women.

As the architect of the Trifecta Light Bed, I'm excited to share its pioneering technology and advancements, distinguishing it from traditional red light therapy beds. Unlike the conventional designs, the Trifecta Light Bed integrates red and near-infrared light. Each spectrum's interaction with the human body varies, allowing the bed to cater to a broader range of user preferences and experiences without specifically stating medical outcomes.

Additionally, the Trifecta Light Bed pioneers a new age of comfort and customization. Its ergonomic design ensures a comfortable user experience during sessions. Moreover, the integrated, cutting-edge cooling system keeps the surface temperature consistently pleasant. In terms of personalization, the Trifecta Light Bed's innovative interface sets it apart, and this unique feature offers the flexibility to modify light intensity and session duration to cater to individual preferences, making each session a unique experience for the user.

Moreover, sustainability has been a guiding principle in the development of the Trifecta Light Bed. Leveraging advanced LED technology, it outperforms traditional incandescent bulbs by a significant margin in energy efficiency, contributing to a more sustainable future. The Trifecta Light Bed, in essence, represents a monumental shift in the design and functionality of light therapy beds. It also symbolizes a delicate marriage of technology and user-focused dcsign, setting a new standard for what light therapy beds can offer to users. The Trifecta does so while remaining conscious of our environmental responsibilities, propelling us into a future where technology meets sustainability.

Choosing the Right Red
Light Therapy Device

With so many different types of red light therapy devices out there, it can be challenging to decide which one is right for your particular needs. Here, we will discuss how to choose the right red light therapy device, including factors to consider, the features of different devices, and where to purchase high-quality products.

I would like to highlight the distinct reasons why this revolutionary light therapy bed outshines others in the market and why it is an excellent addition to your clinic or office. Our Trifecta Light Bed is an embodiment of innovation, standing at the forefront of phototherapeutic technology.

While I refrain from stating explicit medical claims, these modalities cater to a diverse range of user preferences and provide unique user experiences, offering a level of versatility that's truly unmatched.

The design philosophy of the Trifecta Light Bed is centered around the user. The ergonomic design and advanced cooling system ensure a comfortable and enjoyable experience during sessions. These features amplify the appeal of the bed, making it an attractive option for both providers and users. Furthermore, the specially designed interface offers a customizable light therapy experience, allowing for the adjustment of light intensity, frequency, and session duration based on user preferences. This degree of customization is rare in the market, providing a competitive edge for any clinic or office. Additionally, the Trifecta Light Bed is built on a foundation of sustainability and efficiency. The utilization of advanced LED technology significantly outperforms traditional incandescent bulbs in energy consumption. This not only results in lower operating costs but also contributes positively to your environmental footprint. A choice for the Trifecta Light Bed is a choice for a greener future, a statement that resonates with today's environmentally conscious consumers.

Beyond its technical excellence, the Trifecta Light Bed also provides a visually appealing addition to any professional setting. Its sleek design, coupled with the advanced technology within, serves as a reflection of a clinic or office's commitment to incorporating the latest advancements for the benefit of its patrons. Moreover, investing in the Trifecta Light Bed is also a testament to your commitment to providing superior client experiences. The personalized nature of the Trifecta treatments positions your clinic or office as an innovative leader, catering to individual needs and preferences. This focus on personalization will help foster stronger relationships with your clients, enhancing their loyalty and your reputation. The Trifecta Light Bed represents an unparalleled fusion of advanced technology, user-focused design, and sustainability. Its inclusion in your clinic or office signifies your dedication to providing an innovative, personalized, and eco-friendly service, setting you apart from the competition. The Trifecta Light Bed doesn't merely raise the bar; it is the bar. Choosing the Trifecta for your clinic or office is a choice for excellence and a commitment to offering the best to your patrons.

CHAPTER 5

HOW RLT MAY SUPPORT
ANTI-AGING

As we age, our body's natural ability to repair and rejuvenate itself begins to decline, leading to a wide range of physical and aesthetic changes. While there are many anti-aging treatments available that promise to reverse these effects, few are as safe, non-invasive, and effective as red light therapy. As a pioneer in the field of light therapy, I have dedicated my career to exploring the potential benefits of various light-based treatments. A topic of significant interest in contemporary discourse is the application of Red Light Therapy in counteracting the aging process.

Red light therapy, or Photobiomodulation (PBM), involves the exposure of the body to red and Near-Infrared (NIR) light wavelengths, as mentioned in detail. These wavelengths are purported to permeate the skin and tissue, thereby catalyzing cellular processes and augmenting overall health and wellness. The resultant amplified ATP production supports cellular repair, regeneration, and overall function, which can contribute to a rejuvenated appearance.

Red light therapy has clearly demonstrated its ability to enhance blood flow and tissue oxygenation by promoting the release of nitric oxide, which is a potent vasodilator. This improved circulation effectively delivers vital nutrients to the cells while at the same time expelling cellular waste, all of which results in skin that is both healthier and more radiant!

As inflammation is another critical factor in aging and age-related diseases, healing and caring for this issue is essential in skincare treatments. RLT has shown great potential in regulating inflammatory pathways, reducing the production of pro-inflammatory cytokines, and fostering a more balanced immune response. As we age, the production of collagen and elastin, which are crucial proteins in the skin's extracellular matrix, also diminishes, leading to sagging, wrinkles, and other visible signs of aging. However, RLT has been shown to be able to stimulate the production of collagen and elastin, which results in firmer and more resilient skin.

The Trifecta Light Bed is the embodiment of extensive research and development in the field of light therapy, and this advanced device utilizes distinct wavelengths of red and near-infrared light to deliver comprehensive, targeted treatment for anti-aging and holistic wellness.

The Trifecta Light Bed is conceived with comfort, and efficacy as paramount considerations and by integrating

RLT into a holistic anti-aging regimen — which may also encompass a balanced diet, regular exercise, and effective stress management strategies — individuals may promote their health and vitality the body - for years to come!

The Benefits of Red Light Therapy for Anti-Aging

Red light therapy shows promise with a myriad of anti-aging benefits, particularly with regard to mitigating the visible signs of aging. The advantages of this modality include the diminished appearance of wrinkles and fine lines, enhanced skin texture and tone, elevated skin hydration, and accelerated skin healing.

One of the primary mechanisms through which red light therapy attenuates wrinkles and fine lines is the stimulation of collagen production. Collagen is an integral component in maintaining skin resilience and elasticity, and we all experience a decline in its production as we age, resulting in the formation of wrinkles and fine lines. Red light aids in counteracting these manifestations by promoting collagen synthesis, thereby rendering the skin smoother, firmer, and more youthful in appearance. Moreover, red light therapy also augments skin texture and tone, facilitates cellular turnover, and encourages the proliferation of new skin cells. As a result, it serves as an efficacious solution to combat age spots, hyperpigmentation, and other skin irregularities associated with aging.

The 2018 issue of the Journal of Cosmetic Dermatology featured a study titled "Simultaneous application of LED light panels for hydrating facial skin on face and neck" by Weiss and colleagues that explored the benefits of photobiomodulation had 52 people undergo ten sessions of red light therapy, using LED panels that emitted 633 nm wavelength light. The therapy was applied simultaneously to their face and neck, and the researchers measured their skin's hydration levels and hyaluronic acid production before and after the treatment. These results showed that red light therapy resulted in noticeable improvements in skin hydration levels and an increase in the production of hyaluronic acid in the treated areas. Hyaluronic acid is essential for maintaining skin hydration and plumpness as it aids in retaining water in the skin and supporting collagen production. This supplementary hydration aids in alleviating dryness and supports overall skin health. Additionally, red light therapy can also promote skin healing by reducing inflammation and enhancing blood circulation, this being a valuable support for individuals who are undergoing skin treatments, such as laser resurfacing or chemical peels, as it fosters the healing process and stimulates healthy skin regrowth.

It is noteworthy that the effectiveness of red light therapy may vary based on individual characteristics and the specific condition under treatment.

One of the paramount benefits of red light therapy in anti-aging is its non-invasive and safe nature. Unlike other anti-aging modalities such as Botox or fillers that involve needles, incisions, or topical toxins, red light therapy offers an exemplary alternative for individuals seeking to improve their skin's appearance without undergoing invasive procedures.

The Effects of Red Light Therapy on Skin Aging

The inevitable process of skin aging manifests in various dermatological issues, such as sagging, hyperpigmentation, and wrinkle formation. Despite the abundance of skincare products and treatments available in the market, they often fall short of delivering the anticipated results. Nevertheless, red light therapy emerges as a potent, non-invasive treatment promising to stimulate cellular repair and bolster collagen production, consequently enhancing skin texture, elasticity, and firmness.

Studies published in the Journal of Photochemistry and Photobiology (2014) and the Journal of Cosmetic and Laser Therapy (2017) reinforce this mechanism of action, demonstrating significant increases in collagen production and improved skin elasticity and firmness post four weeks of treatment. Additionally, red light therapy also activates fibroblasts, which are the cells directly responsible for collagen production, according to corroborative research. Enhanced blood flow to the skin — another beneficial consequence of red light therapy — also facilitates the delivery of crucial oxygen and nutrients, thereby promoting skin rejuvenation and overall dermal health.

Clinical trials further attest to this treatment's potential to visibly reduce wrinkles and fine lines upon consistent application. For instance, a study published in the Journal of Clinical and Aesthetic Dermatology (2018) reported substantial improvements in the appearance of fine lines, wrinkles, and skin roughness after eight weeks of red light therapy treatment. Known for promoting cellular turnover and exfoliation, red light therapy enhances the skin's texture, rendering it smoother. Additionally, its anti-inflammatory properties posit it as a promising treatment option for acnc-prone skin, effectively mitigating inflammation and reducing uneven skin texture.

Red Light Therapy and Skin Conditions Related to Aging

Extended sun exposure often culminates in the development of age spots; however, red light therapy has demonstrated an ability to improve their appearance. By promoting cellular turnover and reducing melanin production, regular sessions of red light therapy can contribute to a more uniform skin tone and diminish the appearance of age spots. Rosacea, which is a prevalent skin condition typified by facial redness, bumps, and pimples, may also be managed with red light therapy. By increasing blood flow to the affected areas and encouraging cellular regeneration, red light therapy can effectively reduce inflammation. The promotion of natural collagen production and enhanced skin hydration can also lead to more supple and smooth skin, and improve the appearance of age spots, and manage rosacea symptoms and other inflammatory skin conditions.

Red Light Therapy and Hair Loss

Hair loss can be an emotionally distressing experience, often accompanied by a significant reduction in self-esteem and confidence. As we continue to grapple with this pervasive issue, the search for effective treatments remains a top priority in the field of dermatology. One promising approach that has emerged is red light therapy, offering a non-invasive, painless, and safe method to potentially reverse hair loss and stimulate hair growth.

When red and near-infrared light is applied to the scalp, these light wavelengths penetrate the skin and are absorbed by hair follicle cells. These cells, invigorated by the energy imparted by the light, undergo a revitalization that can stimulate hair growth. Again, one of the underlying mechanisms involves the stimulation of the mitochondria within the cells regarding adenosine triphosphate production. ATP is the primary source of energy for cellular processes, and an increase in its production can bolster cell function and proliferation. When applied to hair follicles, this stimulation can potentially reverse miniaturization, a primary contributor to pattern hair loss, and encourage the growth of healthier, fuller hair.

Several studies have corroborated the efficacy of red light therapy in treating hair loss. For instance, a randomized, double-blind study published in the American Journal of Clinical Dermatology in 2014 reported a significant increase in hair density and overall hair growth in subjects who underwent red light therapy compared to a control group. This study illustrates the potential benefits that red light therapy can offer in the realm of hair regrowth, particularly for individuals suffering from androgenetic alopecia.

The application of red light therapy in the field of hair restoration has attracted considerable interest, primarily due to its potential to stimulate hair growth and improve scalp health. An unhealthy scalp can create a formidable barrier to hair growth, leading to complications such as clogged hair follicles, weakened hair strands, and diminished blood circulation. By addressing these issues, red light therapy offers an innovative, non-invasive avenue for treating various hair loss conditions.

Inflammation is also a key contributor to several scalp conditions, including seborrheic dermatitis, psoriasis, and dandruff, which can exacerbate hair loss. Red light therapy, by suppressing the production of cytokines — molecules that promote inflammation — can mitigate the severity of these conditions. The reduction of inflammation subsequently creates a healthier environment for hair follicles, enhancing their capacity to sustain hair growth. Red light therapy also plays a role in sebum regulation. Sebum, an oily substance produced by sebaceous glands in the scalp, is essential for maintaining scalp and hair health. However, excessive sebum can attract bacteria and fungi, leading to scalp infections, such as folliculitis. Red light therapy can modulate sebum production, preventing microbial overgrowth and promoting scalp health, which in turn facilitates hair growth.

Scientific research has increasingly highlighted the efficacy of red light therapy in stimulating hair growth. One particularly illuminating study published in the American Journal of Clinical Dermatology in 2014 reported that low-level laser therapy (LLLT), a variant of red light therapy, significantly increased hair density and growth rate while reducing the severity of hair loss in individuals with androgenetic alopecia, a hereditary form of hair loss. This therapy promotes hair growth by elevating the production of vascular endothelial growth factor (VEGF), a protein crucial to the growth of blood vessels. By increasing blood flow to the hair follicles, more oxygen and nutrients are delivered, promoting hair growth, and it can extend the anagen phase — the active growth stage of the hair cycle — by invigorating cellular activity within hair follicles.

CHAPTER 6

RED LIGHT THERAPY AND
CELLULAR HEALTH

The remarkable world of cellular health is a fascinating field, and the profound impact red light therapy has had in revolutionizing the way we approach wellness and healing is profound. As the developer of the Trifecta Light Bed, I have had the distinct privilege of witnessing firsthand the transformative effects that this modality has had on countless individuals, transcending age, gender, and health conditions. With a foundation in robust scientific research and a commitment to innovation, red light therapy has emerged as a game-changer in the landscape of health and wellness.

To understand the scope of how red light therapy affects the cells, an exploration of the intricacies of cellular health, which is the cornerstone of our overall well-being, is needed. Cellular function plays a critical role in maintaining our bodies' optimal performance, and the disruption of this delicate balance can lead to a plethora of health issues. A closer look at how red light therapy interacts with our cells is needed to understand how it facilitates improved function and fosters an environment conducive to healing and regeneration. There is an extensive body of research that supports the efficacy of red light therapy for a wide array of health concerns, and with each new study, we will gain a deeper understanding of the mechanisms at work, allowing us to refine and enhance our therapeutic approach.

As we navigate the fascinating realm of red light therapy and cellular health, my hope is that you will gain a newfound appreciation for the incredible potential that lies within our cells. Through continued research, innovation, and a dedication to improving the lives of those we serve, red light therapy is poised to redefine the future of health and wellness!

The Function Of Cellular Respiration

To comprehend how red light therapy works, we must understand cellular respiration's fundamental principles. Cells produce energy through a specific process known as "cellular respiration," which occurs mainly in the mitochondria of the cell. The mitochondria, in turn, play an essential role in producing "adenosine triphosphate" (abbreviated to "ATP"). ATP is a molecule that provides energy for other cellular processes; however, environmental stressors, such as pollution or stress from a poor diet or lack of sleep, can interfere with cellular respiration and the production of ATP, leading to cellular damage and dysfunction.

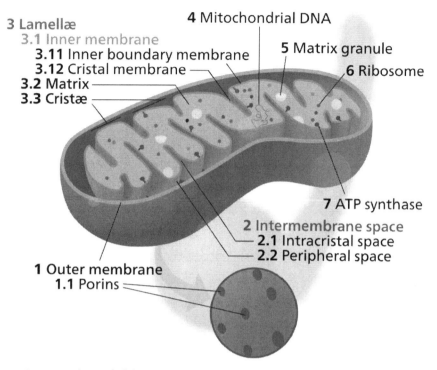

An overview of the anatomical structure of a mitochondrion.
By Kelvinsong, under the Creative Commons License
CC0 1.0 Universal Public Domain.

Red light therapy utilizes red and near-infrared wavelengths of light to penetrate the body and stimulate the mitochondria, which promotes the production of ATP, which in turn improves cellular function and mitochondrial activity. This effect has been shown to increase blood flow, reduce inflammation, and stimulate collagen production, all of which may contribute to better cellular health. In 2020, the Journal of Alzheimer's Disease published a study by Rojas and colleagues titled "Photobiomodulation with Near Infrared Light Mitigates Alzheimer's Disease-Related Pathology in Cerebral Cortex - Evidence from Two Transgenic Mouse Models." This study examined the impact of near-infrared light (NIR) on Alzheimer's disease-related pathology in two different mouse models of the disease. The study exposed mice to 15 minutes of NIR light at a wavelength of 808 nm for four weeks, five days per week. The outcome indicated notable improvements in different aspects of Alzheimer's disease-related pathology, such as lower levels of amyloid-beta protein and reduced inflammation in the brain. Furthermore, the researchers discovered that the brain's mitochondrial activity and ATP production were enhanced with exposure to NIR light.

Mitochondrial Function and ATP Production

The mitochondria are organelles found in almost all eukaryotic cells, which have several fundamental functions in regard to cellular energy production. As mentioned, they are behind the production of the majority of cellular ATP, which is essential for several cellular activities, including maintenance, growth, and repair. The mitochondria produce ATP through a process known as "oxidative phosphorylation," which takes place within the inner mitochondrial membrane. This process involves the transfer of electrons through the electron transport chain, which is a series of protein complexes, also called "ECT." The energy harnessed in this electron transfer is utilized to pump protons (H+) across the inner membrane, creating an electrochemical gradient that is utilized in ATP production, and this process is called chemiosmosis.

Mitochondria play a key role in numerous cellular functions, such as calcium regulation, reactive oxygen species (ROS) generation, neutralization, apoptosis, and metabolism. Additionally, they also act as signaling organelles and participate in cell cycle progression, differentiation, and cell death pathways.

ATP is a high-energy molecule that serves as the primary energy source for almost *all* physiological activities, and the amount of ATP produced by mitochondria depends on the cell's underlying metabolic demand. Under normal physiological conditions, ATP production occurs mainly through oxidative phosphorylation. However, during times of metabolic stress or increased energy demands, non-oxidative pathways, such as glycolysis and creatine phosphate metabolism, can also contribute to ATP production.

Mitochondrial dysfunction has been associated with several pathological conditions, such as cardiovascular diseases, neurodegenerative disorders, and cancer. As red light therapy has been shown to enhance mitochondrial function, this may contribute to its therapeutic effects on symptoms related to these conditions.

Red Light Therapy and Mitochondrial Function

Red light therapy has been found to improve mitochondrial function and, therefore, ATP production through various mechanisms. One example of this is through the increased activity of cytochrome c oxidase, or "CCO," the final protein complex in the electron transport chain that is responsible for transferring electrons to molecular oxygen to create water. It also allows for the absorption of photons by CCO, resulting in a conformational change that increases enzymatic activity, ultimately leading to increased ATP production through oxidative phosphorylation and improved mitochondrial function.

Improved Mitochondrial Membrane Potential

The mitochondrial membrane potential (MMP) is a crucial component of oxidative phosphorylation and a *key* indicator of mitochondrial health. A reduction in MMP can lead to impaired ATP production and mitochondrial dysfunction; however, red light therapy has been found to enhance the activity of mitochondrial enzymes, reduce ROS generation, and improve MMP, which all leads to improved electron transport chain activity, and increased ATP production. Improving mitochondrial function and ATP production is significant for overall cellular energy metabolism and health, and red light therapy has been shown to enhance these vital cellular functions. These findings suggest that red light therapy may have therapeutic potential for mitochondrial dysfunction-related disorders, such as neurodegenerative diseases, metabolic disorders, and aging. Nonetheless, the results represent a promising development in non-invasive, safe, and drug-free therapy options for various conditions involving mitochondrial dysfunction.

The Benefits of Red Light Therapy for Improving Mitochondrial Function

The groundbreaking technology of photobiomodulation, more popularly referred to as red light therapy, capitalizes on the intrinsic healing potential of light. The effect of this light catalyzes cellular regeneration, which effectively augments mitochondrial functionality. Hamblin and colleagues, in their seminal 2019 study published in Biochimica et Biophysica Acta, elucidated the stimulatory effect of this therapy on cytochrome c oxidase - a pivotal enzyme in electron transport and energy production within the mitochondria. Intriguingly, the researchers also observed an augmentation in the number of robust, operationally efficient mitochondria within the cells. This enhancement was attributed to improved mitochondrial respiration and amplified ATP synthesis. Consequently, photobiomodulation is now emerging as a compelling approach to addressing an array of health conditions, particularly those stemming from cellular energy dysfunction.

In a separate investigation, also spearheaded by Hamblin and published in the Journal of Photochemistry and Photobiology, it was found that photobiomodulation can elevate the expression of mitochondrial genes, thereby further optimizing cellular respiration. These groundbreaking findings bear significant implications for individuals grappling with diseases related to the mitochondria or those in pursuit of strategies to boost their cellular metabolic activities. Beyond merely promoting cellular energy production, photobiomodulation has demonstrated great efficacy in mitigating inflammatory responses and fostering tissue regeneration. These attributes further underscore its potential utility in advancing overall health and wellness. Its potential applications extend to individuals with conditions characterized by mitochondrial dysfunction, such as chronic fatigue syndrome, fibromyalgia, and mitochondrial disease. Moreover, the prospects for enhancing athletic performance and catalyzing overall health and wellness render photobiomodulation an exhilarating field of study!

A Reduction of Oxidative Stress

Oxidative stress results from a physiological imbalance where the production of reactive oxygen species (or "ROS") overwhelms the body's natural antioxidant defense mechanisms. Reactive oxygen species are actually free radicals with the potential to damage cellular structures such as proteins, lipids, and DNA. This damage leads to numerous pathological conditions, which include neurodegenerative disorders, cardiovascular diseases, cancer, and aging.

ROS production is tightly regulated by natural antioxidant defense mechanisms in the body, such as enzymes, including superoxide dismutase, catalase, and glutathione peroxidase. An imbalance can occur within this system due to factors like aging, poor diet, exposure to environmental toxins, and chronic inflammation. The resulting reduction in antioxidants increases ROS production, leading to oxidative stress. The accumulation of ROS can further damage the cells, which can cause several pathological conditions in the body.

As an example, oxidative stress has been linked to Alzheimer's disease, Parkinson's disease, cardiovascular disease, diabetes, *and* cancer, among others! In Alzheimer's disease, the accumulation of amyloid-beta protein in the brain can result in oxidative stress, leading to neuronal damage and neurodegeneration. In cardiovascular disease, ROS can damage the endothelium, the inner lining of the blood vessels, leading to the formation of plaques and atherosclerosis. Fortunately, red light therapy has shown great potential for reducing oxidative stress in the body, and many of these studies suggest an exciting new avenue for reducing the negative impact of oxidative stress.

Red Light Therapy and Oxidative Stress Reduction

Red light therapy has garnered considerable attention for its capacity to activate antioxidant enzymes, notably superoxide dismutase, catalase, and glutathione peroxidase, as mentioned. These enzymes orchestrate a cooperative endeavor to neutralize reactive oxygen species (ROS), thereby diminishing oxidative stress within the body. Furthermore, RLT has demonstrated great potential in curtailing ROS production. This intriguing effect has been identified across various cell types, encompassing skin, muscle, and brain cells. One hypothesized mechanism underpinning this effect is photobiomodulation's role in stimulating adenosine triphosphate (ATP) production. An upsurge in ATP production might give rise to a reduction in ROS production, given that ATP is integral to the electron transport chain, a substantial source of ROS.

Red light therapy has also been linked with the stimulation of nitric oxide (NO) production, which is a renowned vasodilator that enhances blood flow. Augmented blood flow, in turn, bolsters the delivery of oxygen and nutrients to the cells, thereby optimizing cellular function and curbing oxidative stress. Oxidative stress, as a physiological imbalance, can pave the way for numerous other pathological conditions, but photobiomodulation has shown promising potential in mitigating oxidative stress through the activation of antioxidant enzymes, the curtailing of ROS production, the stimulation of ATP and NO production, and the enhancement of blood flow.

Evidence of Red Light Therapy for Reducing Oxidative Stress

Numerous studies have investigated the effects of red light therapy on antioxidant enzyme activity, ROS production, and cellular damage caused by oxidative stress. In 2012, Li and colleagues published a study titled "Photobiomodulation with 660-nm and 810-nm light-emitting diode irradiation promotes wound healing in human cells through increased migration and cell proliferation" in Photomedicine and Laser Surgery. They examined how red light therapy can help alleviate cellular damage due to oxidative stress. The researchers applied oxidative stress to human skin fibroblast cells using hydrogen peroxide and then administered red light therapy using LED panels that emit at 660 nm and 810 nm wavelengths. According to the results, red light therapy caused a considerable decrease in damage caused by oxidative stress, including lower levels of ROS production and lipid peroxidation. Moreover, the cells treated with red light therapy showed an increase in antioxidant enzyme activity and glutathione production. This study discovered that red light therapy increased the activity of antioxidant enzymes, such as SOD and catalase, in the cells exposed to oxidative stress. These findings suggest that red light therapy may provide a potential treatment for anti-oxidative stress conditions such as aging, inflammation, and certain types of cancer. Other studies on human skin fibroblasts and myocardial infarction in rats have also reported the efficacy of red light therapy in increasing antioxidant enzyme activities and reducing ROS production. This indicates that red light therapy has the potential to offer numerous benefits, particularly in antioxidant activity and cellular protection. One hypothesis behind red light therapy's mechanism of action proposes that it triggers an increased mitochondrial function, a decrease in ROS production, and an increase in ATP generation. Huang et al.'s study published in the Journal of Biomedical Optics in 2010 thoroughly explored this hypothesis.

Red light therapy's effectiveness may also be due to its ability to use transcription factors, like nuclear factor erythroid 2-related factor 2 (Nrf2), to manage the body's antioxidant defense system. Liang et al.'s study in Free Radical Biology and Medicine, 2017, delves into this hypothesis. Optimal conditions for red light therapy must consider several factors, including wavelength, irradiance, exposure time, and treatment frequency, and patient contextual factors, such as age, skin type, and medical history, should also be considered.

The Regulation of Gene Expressions

The regulation of gene expression is a complicated process that controls the quantity and timing of gene transcription, determining the function and destiny of cells. Poor gene expression has been associated with numerous illnesses, such as cancer, metabolic disorders, and neurodegeneration, and, as a result, regulating gene expression has become a hopeful therapeutic strategy for treating these diseases. Red light therapy has recently gained recognition as a safe and non-invasive way of controlling gene expression, and the mechanism behind regulating gene expression through red light therapy and the scientific evidence that supports its effectiveness is intriguing, to say the least!

The Mechanism of Red Light Therapy-Induced Gene Expression Regulation

Red light therapy works by delivering low-intensity visible, or near-infrared light to the skin or other tissues. This light is, in turn, absorbed by mitochondrial chromophores, like cytochrome c oxidase and flavins. The activation of cellular signaling pathways leads to the activation of transcription factors that can regulate gene expression. Transcription factors are proteins that can bind to DNA and either stimulate or inhibit gene transcription, ultimately affecting the cellular phenotype. Several transcription factors, such as nuclear factor-kappa B (NF-κB), cyclic AMP response element-binding protein (CREB), and heat shock factor (HSF), have been demonstrated to be activated by red light therapy. NF-κB, which is a specific transcription factor, plays a critical role in regulating genes involved in the immune response and inflammation. This transcription factor can promote cell survival by suppressing pro-apoptotic genes and inducing anti-apoptotic genes, like Bcl-2. CREB, another transcription factor, responds to various stimuli like growth factors, stress, and neurotransmitters. It plays a key role in regulating synaptic plasticity, learning, and memory!

While HSF, yet another transcription factor, is activated in response to stress like heat shock or oxidative stress, it is responsible for regulating the expression of heat shock proteins (HSPs) that act as molecular chaperones, protecting cells from damage caused by stress.

One of these genes is fibroblast growth factor 2 (FGF2), which is crucial in promoting angiogenesis and tissue regeneration. Additionally, red light therapy has been shown to be able to increase the expression of matrix metalloproteinases (MMPs), which participate in the extracellular matrix remodeling process during tissue repair. Other studies have demonstrated that red light therapy can enhance the activation of the genes responsible for repairing and regenerating cells, and one of these genes is fibroblast growth factor 2 (FGF2), which is crucial in promoting angiogenesis and tissue regeneration.

Scientific Evidence Supporting the Effectiveness of Red Light Therapy for Gene Expression Regulation

Scientific research has shown that red light therapy can effectively modulate gene expression in various cell types and tissues. One study by Barolet et al., published in the journal Photomedicine and Laser Surgery in 2008, discovered that the therapy can boost collagen expression in human skin fibroblasts, which is crucial for maintaining skin elasticity and integrity, leading to healthier skin. Another investigation conducted by Kim et al., published in the journal Lasers in Medical Science in 2012, found that red light therapy can significantly increase the expression of the genes responsible for producing bone matrix proteins in mesenchymal stem cells taken from rat bone marrow. The therapy was also shown to improve the mineralization capacity of the cells.

In another study by Sommer et al., published in the Journal of Photochemistry and Photobiology B: Biology in 2017, the researchers observed that red light therapy increased the MMPs in cultured human gingival fibroblasts, indicating that it has the potential to enhance wound-healing capabilities by supporting the extracellular matrix's remodeling process. This research has *significant* implications for the use of phototherapy as an alternative therapeutic approach for different wound types.

The use of red light therapy is a promising and safe method for regulating gene expression without invasive procedures. This therapy has been shown to be able to activate various transcription factors and genes related to cellular repair and regeneration, which in turn leads to potential therapeutic benefits.

By harnessing the power of red light therapy, we are not only paving the way for a new era of healthcare but also taking a crucial step toward empowering individuals to take control of their own health and well-being. As the technology behind red light therapy becomes more advanced and accessible, it is my hope that its benefits will be experienced by individuals worldwide, leading to a healthier and happier global population. As we continue to explore the exciting possibilities of red light therapy, it is imperative that we remain dedicated to conducting rigorous scientific research and sharing our findings with the medical community and the general public.

By doing so, we can ensure that red light therapy maintains its momentum as a groundbreaking treatment option and ultimately becomes an integral part of our everyday lives! In conclusion, the future of red light therapy appears to be incredibly promising in its potential to revolutionize the way we approach cellular health and overall wellness.

As the developer of the Trifecta Light Bed, I believe we have only just begun to scratch the surface of what this powerful technology can achieve. Through continuous research and development, we can expect the field of red light therapy to expand and evolve, offering new and innovative treatment methods for a wide range of health conditions. The future of cellular health is bright, and I am honored to be a part of this remarkable development.

CHAPTER 7

CELLULAR ENERGY AND RLT

The production of energy is one of the most vital components of human metabolism and provides power for all of the body's physiological processes, such as cellular growth and repair, physical activity, and the regulation of our body temperature. Two primary metabolic pathways are utilized by the body to generate energy: aerobic metabolism, which requires oxygen, and anaerobic metabolism, which does not.

Aerobic Metabolism

The human body primarily relies on aerobic metabolism to produce energy, which takes place in the mitochondria - the cell's powerhouses. The process of aerobic metabolism includes three stages: glycolysis, the Krebs cycle, and the electron transport chain. Glycolysis takes place in the cytoplasm of the cell and is the first stage of this process. It breaks down glucose into two pyruvate molecules and generates two ATP molecules. The pyruvate molecules then undergo further oxidative breakdown after entering the mitochondria.

The Krebs cycle, or "the citric acid cycle," is the second stage of aerobic metabolism that occurs in the mitochondria's matrix. It comprises a series of enzymatic reactions that convert the pyruvate molecules into carbon dioxide and water. During the Krebs cycle, ATP, NADH, and $FADH_2$ molecules are produced, which provide the necessary energy for the third stage. The electron transport chain is the final stage of aerobic metabolism, taking place in the cristae of the mitochondria. In this stage, redox reactions transfer electrons from NADH and $FADH_2$ molecules to oxygen molecules, producing energy in the form of ATP. Oxygen is a crucial element in this stage, as it acts as the final electron acceptor, facilitating the efficient production of energy.

The respiratory system plays a critical role in aerobic metabolism by delivering oxygen to the cells. Through inhalation, oxygen reaches the lungs and diffuses into the bloodstream, binding to hemoglobin. Hemoglobin transports oxygen to the cells, where it combines with other molecules to produce energy through aerobic metabolism.

Anaerobic Metabolism

When there is a scarcity of oxygen, anaerobic metabolism initiates as a metabolic pathway. This pathway is typically used during intense exercise or hypoxia, where energy demand is high and the oxygen supply is limited. There are two types of anaerobic metabolism, namely lactate fermentation and the phosphagen system. Lactate fermentation happens in the cytoplasm of the cell. During this process, glucose breaks down into pyruvate, which is then converted into lactate. Though this process produces a small amount of ATP, it is less efficient than aerobic metabolism. The accumulation of lactate in the body leads to lactate acidosis, which causes fatigue and muscle soreness when energy demand exceeds oxygen supply.

On the other hand, the phosphagen system is a metabolic pathway that occurs in muscle cells. It involves breaking down creatine phosphate to produce energy. This pathway is used in situations where energy demand is high but brief, such as during a short burst of high-intensity exercise. Despite producing a small amount of ATP, the phosphagen system is efficient in providing immediate energy.

The Limitations of Energy Production

The human body has efficient metabolic pathways to generate energy, but there are restrictions to energy production due to the availability of oxygen. If there is a shortage of oxygen, aerobic metabolism cannot happen, and the body relies on anaerobic metabolism, which is not as effective. Moreover, age and diseases can hinder the body's energy production capability. As we grow older, our metabolism slows down, and our energy production capacity decreases. Illnesses like cancer and diabetes can also disrupt energy production by modifying metabolic pathways or interfering with oxygen distribution.

Energy production is crucial to human metabolism as it fuels physiological processes. However, when energy production becomes limited, it can result in fatigue and contribute to the development of various diseases. Thus, understanding the various stages of energy production and their limitations may help optimize and manage energy production effectively.

The Role of ATP in Energy Transfer

As already touched upon, adenosine triphosphate (ATP) plays a critical role in energy metabolism, serving as the primary source of energy for cellular processes in living organisms. ATP is produced through different metabolic pathways and utilized in various physiological processes. The most significant pathway is oxidative phosphorylation, which occurs in the mitochondria. During this process, electrons move through the mitochondrial electron transport chain and create a proton gradient, resulting in ATP synthesis. Another pathway, substrate-level phosphorylation, directly transfers phosphate groups to ADP from high-energy molecules during glycolysis or the citric acid cycle. In bacteria and archaea, ATP synthesis occurs through chemiosmotic coupling, which links ion gradient formation with ATP synthesis across the cell membrane.

ATP is absolutely instrumental in a variety of physiological processes, such as muscle contraction, nerve impulse transmission, and protein synthesis. During muscle contraction, ATP hydrolysis is responsible for generating the required energy. As the contraction occurs, ATP breaks down into Adenosine Diphosphate and inorganic phosphate, releasing energy utilized by myosin heads to generate force and movement. In nerve impulse transmission, ATP also plays a critical role. Once a nerve impulse reaches the synaptic terminal, ATP is released, activating receptors on the postsynaptic membrane, thus enabling the impulse to cross the synapse. ATP is also considered indispensable in protein synthesis, as it provides the energy necessary for linking amino acids through peptide bonds, and such peptide bond formation requires energy, which is supplied by ATP hydrolysis.

ATP Maintenance and Depletion

The human body has a highly efficient system for regulating ATP levels: these levels are continuously replenished through various mechanisms, as discussed earlier. Additionally, the body also stores "ATP reserves" via what is known as the ATP-PCr system, which provides energy for shorter, high-intensity activities such as sprinting, jumping, and weightlifting. When ATP levels become depleted, it can lead to severe consequences such as muscle weakness, fatigue, and even cellular death! In such cases, the body turns to alternative energy sources such as glucose and fatty acids, which causes the metabolism to shift towards anaerobic respiration. This leads to the accumulation of lactic acid, which causes fatigue, and ATP depletion is a hallmark of many degenerative diseases. It is a crucial element of energy metabolism and a significant signaling molecule in cellular processes and plays a critical role in muscle contraction, nerve impulse transmission, and protein synthesis.

Although the body has a well-organized mechanism for producing and maintaining ATP levels, its depletion can have serious consequences!

The Mechanisms of Red Light Therapy in Enhancing Energy Production

As covered earlier in the book, the mitochondria serve as the main source of energy production for the cell. As mentioned earlier, they are crucial in facilitating the electron transport chain, which produces ATP. As electrons move through various respiratory enzyme complexes, oxygen ultimately becomes the final electron acceptor. This creates a proton motive force across the inner mitochondrial membrane, which powers ATP synthase to convert ADP and phosphate into ATP.

Electron Transport Chain and Cytochrome c Oxidase:

Cytochrome c oxidase is the enzyme responsible for the final step in the electron transport chain. It is located in the inner mitochondrial membrane and accepts electrons from cytochrome c, passing them on to oxygen, which is then reduced to water. This reaction is vital for the production of adenosine triphosphate as it generates a proton motive force used by ATP synthase to produce ATP.

Red light therapy has been shown to *increase* the activity of cytochrome c oxidase, and this effect is hypothesized to be due to the absorption of photons by the enzyme, which activates it and increases its activity. This activation is thought to occur via the chromophore heme, which is present in cytochrome c oxidase. The absorption of red and near-infrared light by heme can lead to a conformational change in the enzyme and an increase in its activity. Additionally, red light therapy leads to an increase in the production of nitric oxide, which also stimulates cytochrome c oxidase activity.

Stimulation of the Production of New Mitochondria:

Red light therapy has also been shown to stimulate the production of *new* mitochondria, which is a process known as "mitochondrial biogenesis." This process involves the activation of various signaling pathways, such as the peroxisome proliferator-activated receptor gamma co-activator 1-alpha (PGC-1α) pathway, which promotes the expression of genes involved in mitochondrial biogenesis. PGC-1α is thought to be activated by red light therapy through the activation of AMP-activated protein kinase (AMPK) and sirtuins.

Enhanced Mitochondrial Function:

Furthermore, red and near-infrared light has been shown to enhance mitochondrial function. This effect is thought to be due to the increased activity of cytochrome c oxidase, which enhances the efficiency of the electron transport chain, leading to increased ATP production. Additionally, this therapy can increase the expression of genes involved in mitochondrial function, such as those encoding mitochondrial uncoupling proteins (UCPs), leading to improved mitochondrial efficiency.

Clinical Applications of Red Light Therapy
for Enhancing Energy Production

The ability of red light therapy to enhance energy production has significant clinical applications; It has been shown to improve muscle performance, reduce muscle fatigue, and improve exercise tolerance. Red light therapy has also been shown to improve cognitive function and reduce the symptoms of neurodegenerative diseases such as Alzheimer's disease. Additionally, it has been shown to improve wound healing, as increased energy production can enhance tissue regeneration.

Millions of Americans experience fatigue on a daily basis due to various factors such as stress, illness, lack of sleep, and poor nutrition. Some individuals struggle with chronic fatigue, which can greatly affect their quality of life. Fortunately, red light therapy has emerged as a promising treatment option for fatigue. This non-invasive procedure utilizes red light to promote cellular activity and healing.

According to research conducted by Lane et al., the use of red light therapy was found to have a significant impact on the expression of cytochrome c oxidase in skeletal muscle cells, resulting in an improvement in muscle performance and a reduction of muscle fatigue. Additionally, a separate study by Wang et al., published in the journal Biochimica et Biophysica Acta (BBA) - General Subjects in 2017, discovered that RLT enhanced mitochondrial respiration and increased ATP production in human skin cells. These findings indicate that RLT can be an effective treatment option for improving mitochondrial function while reducing fatigue.

The Reduction Of Inflammation

Fatigue is a common problem that can arise from a variety of factors, such as stress, illness, or injury. These factors can lead to chronic inflammation, which can damage cells and ultimately contribute to fatigue. However, one promising solution to this issue is red light therapy, and research has shown that red light therapy can help reduce inflammation and activate anti-inflammatory pathways in the body. By doing so, RLT has the potential to prevent cellular damage and boost energy levels. For instance, Avni et al. found that RLT was effective in reducing inflammation, improving joint function, and reducing pain in patients with rheumatoid arthritis. Similarly, Huang et al. discovered that RLT was also effective in reducing inflammation and oxidative stress in cells that were exposed to ultraviolet radiation. In yet another study published in the Journal of Biomedical Optics 2015, it was found that exposing cells to red and NIR light increased the activity of CCO, leading to a subsequent increase in ATP production.

Other studies have additionally demonstrated that red light therapy may enhance energy metabolism by boosting oxygen consumption and decreasing oxidative stress; Oxygen is indispensable to cellular respiration, the process that generates energy in our cells. According to a research paper published in the Journal of Photochemistry and Photobiology B: Biology, red light exposure elevates cellular oxygen consumption, leading to increased ATP production.

CHAPTER 8

RED LIGHT THERAPY
AND PAIN RELIEF

In the world of contemporary health therapies, Red Light Therapy has emerged as a promising non-invasive treatment modality, especially for its potential in pain relief. As the developer of the Trifecta Light Bed, an innovative red light therapy device, I aim to contribute to this ongoing dialogue surrounding the efficacy and mechanism of RLT for pain management. Chronic pain is often associated with conditions such as osteoarthritis, fibromyalgia, and neuropathy and significantly impedes the quality of life for millions worldwide.

While conventional pain management strategies often rely on pharmacological interventions, these treatments can potentially lead to unwanted side effects and dependency issues. This is where RLT, with its minimal side effects, becomes an attractive alternative. RLT operates within the spectrum of light therapy and utilizes wavelengths in the range of 630-660 nm (red light) and 810-1000 nm (near-infrared light). The ability of RLT to penetrate the skin and underlying tissues allows it to act at the cellular level. Essentially, the mitochondria within cells absorb the red and near-infrared light, leading to increased production of adenosine triphosphate (ATP), the energy currency of cells. Enhanced ATP production is believed to accelerate cellular repair and regeneration, reduce inflammation, and alleviate pain.

A multitude of clinical studies substantiates the analgesic properties of red light therapy. For instance, a meta-analysis disseminated in the 2017 edition of Pain Research and Treatment proposed that RLT could be instrumental in managing chronic musculoskeletal pain. Concurrently, a study published in the Journal of Physical Therapy Science in 2016 pointed to RLT's potential to enhance functionality and relieve pain in individuals grappling with knee osteoarthritis. This promising body of evidence strengthens the case for RLT as a promising frontier for pain mitigation. However, it is crucial to acknowledge that more extensive and rigorous clinical trials are necessary for a thorough comprehension of RLT's range and efficacy.

In the context of chronic conditions such as osteoarthritis, lower back pain, fibromyalgia, and Temporomandibular Disorder (TMD), RLT has shown notable efficacy in pain alleviation. For instance, a study spearheaded by Chow et al. published in the journal Pain Research & Management in 2006 established that patients suffering from chronic joint disorders, inclusive of osteoarthritis, witnessed an enhancement in function and a decrease in pain intensity following RLT. Similarly, Toma et al.'s study, published in the journal Lasers in Medical Science in 2018, found significant pain abatement in patients with lower back pain who received RLT. These findings collectively indicate that RLT could potentially serve as a valuable therapeutic tool for individuals suffering from chronic pain conditions.

The Anti-Inflammatory Effects
of Red Light Therapy

Inflammation is a natural physiological response to injury, infection, or stress. However, persistent inflammation can precipitate tissue damage and engender chronic pain. Several studies have demonstrated that red light therapy can modulate inflammation by regulating the activity of immune cells, including macrophages and lymphocytes. These cells generate cytokines - signaling molecules integral to inflammation, immune response, and tissue repair.

Research spearheaded by Hamblin et al., published in the journal "Photomedicine and Laser Surgery," unveiled that RLT enhances the production of anti-inflammatory cytokines such as interleukin-10, while simultaneously attenuating the levels of pro-inflammatory cytokines, including interleukin-1 beta and tumor necrosis factor-alpha. This dual action is conjectured to foster a balanced immune response, leading to pain reduction and enhanced healing. Moreover, it has been shown to mitigate oxidative stress instigated by free radicals, which can inflict cellular damage on proteins, lipids, and DNA, thereby leading to chronic diseases and inflammation. RLT is capable of amplifying the activity of antioxidant enzymes, including superoxide dismutase and catalase, which neutralize free radicals and prevent cellular damage.

Beyond its anti-inflammatory impacts, red and near-infrared light may also alleviate pain sensation, functioning as an analgesic. Pain is a multifaceted process involving various pathways and receptors in the nervous system. RLT can modulate these pathways by escalating the release of natural analgesics like endorphins and other neurotransmitters. Recent research unveiled that RLT can enhance the expression of mu-opioid receptors, the primary receptors for endorphins. This amplifies the analgesic impact of endorphins and diminishes pain perception.

By increasing the production of nitric oxide, RLT can promote better blood flow to the affected area, reducing muscle tension and enhancing the delivery of oxygen and nutrients to the tissues. This, in turn, supports healing and reduces the sensation of pain. Moreover, red light therapy can inhibit the activity of pain receptors such as TRPV1 and TRPA1, which are known to become overactive in response to injury or inflammation, leading to hypersensitivity and chronic pain.

By modulating their activity and reducing their expression, red light therapy can effectively desensitize these receptors and alleviate the pain sensation. Taken together, these findings suggest that red light therapy is a highly effective therapeutic intervention for managing pain.

Improved Blood Flow

Among the numerous benefits conferred by red light therapy, its capacity to enhance blood flow stands as a significant advantage. Scientific research has revealed that red and near-infrared light can instigate the release of nitric oxide, a molecule paramount for relaxing blood vessels and augmenting blood flow. Regulating blood pressure, attenuating inflammation, and improving systemic circulation are critical functions of nitric oxide. By stimulating nitric oxide production, RLT can efficiently enhance the delivery of oxygen and nutrients to cells throughout the organism. A study done by published by Mayr et al., 2013, which was disseminated in the Journal of the American Geriatrics Society, reported that individuals subjected to RLT exhibited a considerable increase in blood flow compared to those without exposure to this therapy. The study deduced that RLT harbors the potential to serve as an effective therapeutic intervention for enhancing blood flow, particularly in elderly patients afflicted with peripheral artery disease.

In addition to improving blood flow, RLT is also capable of augmenting tissue oxygenation, which is achieved via an upsurge in adenosine triphosphate (ATP) production, which, in turn, bolsters cellular function and facilitates a more efficient transfer of oxygen from the bloodstream to tissues. Enhanced tissue oxygenation is a cornerstone of the healing process, as it fosters the growth of new blood vessels and tissues. This feature has been demonstrated to be notably efficacious in improving tissue oxygenation in patients with chronic wounds. A study published in the International Wound Journal, conducted by Schubert and colleagues, 2016, affirmed that RLT significantly improved oxygen saturation and wound healing in patients suffering from chronic leg ulcers.

Furthermore, this therapy has been found to stimulate the formation of new blood vessels, a process crucial for tissue repair and regeneration known as angiogenesis. Scientific research supports that RLT can induce angiogenesis by enhancing the production of growth factors and cytokines necessary for blood vessel formation; as per a review article in the Journal of Photochemistry and Photobiology B: Biology by Hamblin and colleagues, 2017, RLT could serve as a therapeutic intervention for promoting angiogenesis and tissue repair across a wide array of medical conditions.

Applications of Red Light Therapy for Pain Relief

Arthritis is characterized by joint inflammation that leads to stiffness and pain and significantly hampers mobility. It is a pervasive condition. As mentioned, red light acts by catalyzing the production of adenosine triphosphate, a molecule integral to cellular energy production. The mitochondria assimilate the light energy, thus stimulating ATP production. Consequently, elevated ATP levels endorse cellular repair and regeneration, attenuating inflammation and joint pain. Several clinical studies have scrutinized the efficacy of RLT in providing relief from arthritis pain, and a randomized placebo-controlled study published in the journal Lasers in Medical Science, in 2014, by Al Rashoud and colleagues observed individuals with knee osteoarthritis undergoing RLT thrice a week over a month, noting a considerable reduction in pain and stiffness, complemented by improved joint mobility. Analogous results were also reported in a study focusing on rheumatoid arthritis patients.

RLT in Sports Medicine:
Treating Injuries

The application of red light therapy in sports medicine for the treatment of varied injuries, including strains, sprains, and muscle soreness, is widespread. red and near-infrared light has been studied extensively and shown to offer pain relief, accelerate tissue repair, and curtail inflammation. RLT functions by enhancing collagen production, a protein critical for new tissue growth in the body. Injuries tend to deplete collagen levels, but RLT can stimulate its production, leading to quicker healing times. Moreover, it augments blood flow, facilitating the delivery of essential nutrients and oxygen to the affected area, promoting healing, and reducing inflammation. RLT is a safe therapeutic solution with no known adverse effects, making it an invaluable tool for individuals grappling with pain from various conditions, including arthritis and sports injuries.

RLT and Postoperative Pain Management

Unmanaged postoperative pain following surgical procedures can lead to extended recovery periods, heightened risk of infections, and diminished quality of life, making it a significant concern. Traditional pain management techniques, such as opioid medications, often come with several side effects, including addiction, constipation, nausea, and confusion. Recently, researchers have been investigating alternative treatment approaches, leading to the advent of RLT as a promising solution. RLT can reduce inflammation, facilitate tissue healing, and alleviate pain by stimulating the production of ATP, the primary source of cellular energy. Furthermore, RLT has been demonstrated to induce the production of endorphins, natural painkillers synthesized by the body, thus reducing reliance on opioid pain medications.

Promoted Tissue Healing with RLT

The recuperation process post-surgery necessitates efficient tissue healing. A study done by Hamblin and colleagues that was published in the journal Photobiomodulation, Photomedicine, and Laser Surgery in 2017 suggests red and near-infrared light capabilities promote healing by amplifying collagen production, a crucial protein for tissue growth and repair. Patients receiving RLT reported less incision pain and reduced scar tissue formation compared to those who did not receive the therapy. These findings hint at RLT's potential to hasten the healing process and improve recovery rates, particularly in cesarean delivery patients. This study has significant implications for maternal health and contributes to the burgeoning literature exploring the benefits of alternative healing methods in mainstream medicine. Pain relief constitutes the most vital aspect of postoperative care.

RLT has also been shown to alleviate pain by stimulating endorphin production, the body's natural painkillers. It can complement traditional pain management techniques, such as opioids, which often come with adverse side effects.

Scientific Evidence for Red Light Therapy in Pain Relief

Pain is a universal experience linked to a myriad of conditions such as arthritis, back pain, neuropathic pain, and sports injuries, and it can trigger both physical and emotional discomfort, mood alterations, and a diminished quality of life. Red light therapy) has risen to prominence in the field of pain management. Numerous clinical trials have endeavored to assess the efficacy of RLT in pain relief, and a study conducted by Zhang et al. (2020) involving 103 patients diagnosed with knee osteoarthritis randomly assigned the participants to receive either authentic or sham RLT over a duration of four weeks. The results indicated that the RLT cohort exhibited significant enhancements in pain intensity, stiffness, and physical function when compared to the sham cohort.

Similarly, Gurgen et al. (2020) engaged 34 patients suffering from plantar fasciitis in a study, assigning them to either RLT or sham therapy over a two-week period. Post-treatment, the RLT group manifested a notable reduction in pain and a marked functional enhancement relative to the sham group.

The therapeutic prowess of RLT extends to patients grappling with neuropathic pain as well. Barolet et al. (2016) initiated a pilot study involving 24 patients afflicted with neuropathic pain. The treatment regimen entailed RLT exposure thrice weekly over a four-week span. Both pain intensity and quality of life exhibited significant improvements in the RLT group when contrasted with the baseline assessment.

In yet another pivotal study orchestrated by Dima et al. (2019), 60 patients with chronic low back pain were enrolled. These individuals received either RLT or a placebo therapy over a period of six weeks. The cohort subjected to RLT showcased a substantial reduction in both pain intensity and disability compared to the placebo cohort.

Systematic Reviews and Meta-Analyses on RLT's Effectiveness in Pain Relief

Several comprehensive reviews and analyses have been conducted on RLT's effectiveness in alleviating pain. A study by Huang et al. (2018) observed six Randomized Controlled Trials (RCTs) involving 377 patients diagnosed with chronic musculoskeletal pain, concluding that RLT exerted moderate pain relief effects with no adverse events reported. A different review conducted by Tafur et al. (2016) analyzed 18 RCTs investigating RLT for various conditions, including musculoskeletal pain, skin wounds, and neuropathic pain. The authors inferred that RLT exerted positive effects on pain relief and functional improvement. Furthermore, systematic reviews have been conducted to examine the mechanism of action of RLT in pain relief. Ferraresi et al. (2015) reviewed 42 studies investigating the molecular and cellular effects of RLT, finding that it mitigated oxidative stress and inflammation, and bolstered mitochondrial function. Such empirical findings continue to underscore the powerful therapeutic potential of photobiomodulation in managing diverse types of pain.

As the developer behind the Trifecta Light Bed, I have spent considerable time immersed in the intricacies of RLT; it is a fascinating domain offering expansive therapeutic possibilities. This remarkable modality leverages the principles of photobiomodulation, utilizing specific wavelengths of light to stimulate cellular function, enhance healing, and alleviate pain.

While we have made strides in understanding the cellular and molecular mechanisms of RLT, much remains to be discovered. Future research should strive to further elucidate the precise pathways through which RLT exerts its effects and identify the specific targets involved. This deeper understanding will not only enhance our appreciation of RLT's mechanisms of action but also guide the development of more targeted and effective treatment strategies.

As the developer of the groundbreaking technology of the Trifecta Light Bed, I have witnessed firsthand the incredible results this therapy can achieve in improving the quality of life for countless individuals! Our world is currently facing an unprecedented crisis in pain management, with millions of people suffering from chronic pain and held in the grip of the Opioid crisis. The need for effective, non-invasive, and *drug-free* solutions has never been more urgent.

Red light therapy, and in particular the Trifecta Light Bed, may offer hope for millions of individuals that are seeking a more natural way of attaining relief from their pain. As we move forward, I am confident that our continued research and innovation will only strengthen the case for red light therapy as a cornerstone of modern pain management. My team and I are committed to pushing the boundaries of what is possible by harnessing the power of red light to create a brighter, pain-free future for all.

CHAPTER 9

SKIN HEALTH AND THE
BENEFITS OF RLT

I have had the unique privilege of delving into the profound implications of red light therapy across various health applications and studying its incredible benefits first-hand. The quest for maintaining youthful and healthy skin has led to the development of various skin care regimens and treatments. Traditionally, these protocols involved the use of topical treatments, exfoliants, and moisturizers. However, recent advancements in the field of skin care have opened up new avenues for promoting skin health, one of which is red light therapy.

As the developer of the Trifecta Light Bed, I am excited to share the numerous benefits of red light therapy and its potential to transform skin rejuvenation procedures. Incorporating red light therapy into a skin care regimen can provide numerous benefits, particularly when it comes to skin rejuvenation. As we age, our skin cells begin to lose their ability to function optimally, leading to the appearance of fine lines, wrinkles, and other signs of aging. Red light therapy has been shown to stimulate the production of collagen and elastin – two essential proteins responsible for maintaining skin elasticity and firmness.

By increasing the production of these proteins, red light therapy can effectively reduce the appearance of wrinkles and promote a more youthful complexion. Integrating red light therapy into a skincare routine is simple with the Trifecta Light Bed. Treatment sessions typically last between 10 to 20 minutes and can be performed multiple times per week, depending on the individual's skin care goals and needs. During a session, the individual lies on the bed, which emits red and near-infrared light onto the skin. The treatment is painless, non-invasive, and requires no downtime, allowing individuals to easily incorporate it into their existing skin care regimen.

Red light therapy offers promising support to traditional skin care treatments and has the potential to greatly improve overall skin health and appearance. By incorporating RLT into a regular skincare routine, individuals can effectively stimulate collagen production, improve skin tone and texture, reduce inflammation, and promote faster healing – all of which contribute to a more youthful and radiant complexion. Among the most compelling of these is the potential of RLT to promote skin health. As previously discussed, RLT is based on the principles of photobiomodulation and employs specific wavelengths of light to influence cellular behavior. The therapy offers many benefits regarding skin health, ranging from enhanced wound healing to improved complexion and skin tone. One of the primary mechanisms underlying these advantages involves the stimulation of fibroblasts, which are cells that are responsible for collagen production.

This reduction of collagen as we age manifests as fine lines, wrinkles, and sagging skin. RLT has demonstrated a powerful capacity to stimulate collagen production, leading to improvements in skin texture, tone, and radiance. The facilitation of collagen synthesis by RLT operates primarily through the activation of fibroblasts, the cells responsible for collagen and extracellular matrix protein production. These proteins provide essential structural reinforcement to the skin. RLT induces a minor inflammatory response in fibroblasts, leading to the release of specific growth factors that spur collagen and elastin synthesis. A study published in the Journal of Photomedicine and Laser Surgery by Wunsch and colleagues, 2014, documented significant improvements in skin elasticity and firmness among 30 participants aged 30-60 following 12 weeks of RLT. This study also indicated a marked reduction in wrinkles and fine lines.

Additionally, while inflammation is a natural bodily response to injury or infection, chronic inflammation can detrimentally affect skin health, contributing to conditions like eczema, psoriasis, and acne. Red light has demonstrated notable anti-inflammatory effects in mitigating the production of pro-inflammatory cytokines and enhancing the release of their anti-inflammatory counterparts. These actions can alleviate skin redness, swelling, and irritation, and a study in the Journal of Investigative Dermatology in 2017 by Kim and colleagues, found that

RLT diminished inflammation in patients with chronic rosacea.

As mentioned in great detail, red and near-infrared light also promotes mitochondrial function, resulting in increased ATP generation, which can additionally lead to skin rejuvenation and improve cellular turnover. It has also been found to enhance skin blood flow, thus delivering more oxygen and nutrients to the skin, which fosters the removal of toxins.

RLT has furthermore been shown to speed up wound healing by stimulating collagen production and encouraging angiogenesis, which is the new blood vessel formation process. Oxidative stress is characterized by an imbalance between the reactive oxygen species production and the body's capability to neutralize them, which can lead to cellular and tissue damage and so cause aging and disease. When ROS accumulate in the skin, they tend to induce oxidative damage, which results in wrinkles, fine lines, hyperpigmentation, and other aging signs.

Furthermore, UV radiation from sun exposure, along with pollution, smoking, alcohol consumption, and a poor diet, significantly contribute to skin oxidative stress. RLT has demonstrated the capacity to mitigate oxidative stress in the skin by activating antioxidant enzymes that neutralize free radicals, thereby reducing their damaging effects on skin cells. Studies have also shown that RLT can enhance the activity of superoxide dismutase (SOD), which is a potent antioxidant enzyme.

Applications of Red Light Therapy for Skin Health

Acne is a prevalent skin condition which impacts millions of individuals globally. Multiple factors, including excessive sebum production, hormonal fluctuations, and bacterial proliferation on the skin, contribute to its onset. Red light has demonstrated efficacy in acne treatment by diminishing inflammation, modulating sebum production, and eradicating acne-inducing bacteria. RLT functions by penetrating the skin to stimulate cellular activity, and it mitigates inflammation and accelerates healing by enhancing blood flow to the treatment site. Significantly, RLT also helps regulate sebum production, which is a crucial factor in acne pathogenesis.

By curtailing excessive sebum production, red and near-infrared light aids in averting pore blockage and subsequent acne formation. Additionally, it can effectively neutralize acne-promoting bacteria, such as Propionibacterium acnes. This bacterium thrives in an oxygen-deficient environment, the precise conditions created during acne development. RLT penetrates the skin and eliminates the bacteria by releasing singlet oxygen molecules, which oxidize the bacterial cell wall, rendering them innocuous. Empirical evidence supports the use of RLT in acne management. A 2016 study published in the Journal of Cosmetic and Laser Therapy, conducted by Lee and colleagues, reported a reduction in acne lesion count by up to 77% following three monthly RLT sessions. In another study, the combination of RLT with topical acne medication outperformed the use of medication alone in reducing acne.

Red Light Therapy for Psoriasis and Other Skin Conditions

Psoriasis, a chronic autoimmune disease, presents with dry, itchy, and scaly skin patches. Red light therapy demonstrates potential in treating psoriasis by attenuating inflammation, invigorating cellular activity, and enhancing overall skin health.

As mentioned, RLT operates by penetrating the skin and mitigating inflammation via the generation of singlet oxygen molecules, which alleviate swelling and redness. RLT also modulates the immune response, which is a pivotal aspect of psoriasis treatment, as well. By invigorating cellular activity, RLT fosters healthy skin growth, reduces scaly patches, and prevents the formation of new ones. Several skin conditions, including psoriasis, eczema, and rosacea, can inflict *significant* discomfort and impair an individual's quality of life.

A particular study published in Clinical and Experimental Dermatology in 2013, titled "Effectiveness of red light therapy for the treatment of psoriasis: a systematic review and meta-analysis," reviewed 13 randomized controlled trials conducted between 2000 and 2012. The authors of this study, H.S. Huang et al., found that red light therapy significantly improved psoriasis symptoms compared to placebo treatment. Additionally, they found that red light therapy was well-tolerated and had no significant adverse effects. In a more recent study published in Photobiomodulation, Photomedicine, and Laser Surgery in 2020, titled "Low-Level Light Therapy for Psoriasis: A Systematic Review and Meta-Analysis," the authors, S. Liu et al., also conducted a meta-analysis of randomized controlled trials. The study found that red light therapy significantly improved psoriasis symptoms, with no significant adverse events reported.

Scientific Evidence for Red Light Therapy in Skin Health

Red light therapy has gained recognition in the scientific community and the beauty industry as an innovative, safe, and effective treatment for a range of skin conditions. By utilizing wavelengths of red light, RLT penetrates the skin's surface, catalyzing an array of physiological processes that collectively enhance skin health. The amount of scientific literature on RLT has been growing rapidly in recent years, showing empirical evidence that supports its effectiveness in various dermatological applications. Here, we will analyze the scientific evidence highlighting the use of RLT in the management of acne and the reversal of aging signs.

Acne is a very pervasive skin affliction that is not confined to any age group. The proposition of RLT as a therapeutic modality for acne has garnered considerable attention, supported by a substantial body of research affirming its effectiveness. Clinical investigations have reported that RLT can reduce inflammation, curtail sebum production, and mitigate the extent of acne lesions. A notable study by Lee et al., published in the Journal of Investigative Dermatology in 2007, demonstrated a significant reduction in acne lesions post-RLT treatment spanning 12 weeks - inflammatory acne lesions diminished by 67%, and non-inflammatory acne lesions declined by 34%. This reduction can be credited to the RLT's capacity to increase blood circulation and stimulate collagen synthesis, which together rejuvenates the skin, thereby alleviating inflammation and reducing the onset of new acne lesions.

In terms of anti-aging interventions, RLT has been increasingly adopted due to its potential to reverse the signs of aging and enhance overall skin aesthetics. Multiple clinical trials have corroborated these claims, establishing that RLT can diminish the manifestation of fine lines, wrinkles, and other aging signs. A seminal study by Wunsch and Matuschka, published in the journal Laser Therapy in 2014, evidenced a remarkable increase of 50% in the density of collagen fibers in the skin following 12 weeks of RLT treatment.

This amplified collagen synthesis results in enhanced skin elasticity, thereby reducing fine lines and wrinkles. Furthermore, RLT has been shown to improve the overall texture and tone of the skin, imparting a more youthful, radiant complexion. This can be attributed to RLT's role in increasing cutaneous blood flow, which nourishes the skin and stimulates healthy cellular growth. In terms of safety considerations, RLT represents a scientifically validated, safe, and effective skincare option. Its proven proficiency in reducing inflammation, sebum production, and acne lesions renders it a compelling treatment alternative for individuals grappling with acne. Additionally, its ability to boost collagen production and skin elasticity positions it as a promising solution for reversing the signs of aging and enhancing overall skin health.

The Trifecta Light Bed can play a pivotal role in revolutionizing the way skin health is approached. The advancements we have made in this field will undoubtedly continue to grow, paving the way for groundbreaking innovations that will further enhance the benefits of red light therapy for all. Our research has only scratched the surface of the potential applications of red light therapy, and I am excited to further explore and uncover new possibilities. The Trifecta is a testament to ingenuity, and I am proud to be at the forefront of this cutting-edge technology along with my team. With every success we achieve and every milestone we surpass, we move closer to realizing a world where red light therapy is an integral part of maintaining the health and vitality of skincare.

CHAPTER 10

RED LIGHT THERAPY AND
MUSCLE RECOVERY

Muscle recovery is a fundamental aspect of any individual's physical well-being, be it an athlete pushing their limits or a fitness enthusiast striving for progress. Traditionally, the methods employed for muscle recovery have been limited in their efficacy and often accompanied by notable downtime. However, with the advent of red light therapy, a promising new avenue has emerged, heralding a paradigm shift in how we approach muscle recuperation.

Red and near-infrared light has demonstrated remarkable potential in promoting muscle recovery and reducing the time required for tissue repair, and by penetrating deep into the layers of our musculature, red light stimulates vital cellular processes, triggering a cascade of beneficial effects that expedite healing and enhance overall muscle resilience.

Inflammation is the body's natural response to injury, infection, or tissue damage. However, as mentioned earlier, the persistence of inflammation can lead to chronic diseases and is often the underlying cause of muscle soreness and fatigue. RLT offers notable anti-inflammatory effects by reducing cytokine production and increasing the presence of anti-inflammatory cytokines. Cytokines are crucial proteins within the immune system that play a pivotal role in the body's response to inflammation. When the body experiences injury or stress, cytokines are released to initiate an inflammatory response. However, *excessive* cytokine production can result in prolonged inflammation and lead to tissue damage and delayed recovery. RLT, on the other hand, has been observed to mitigate inflammation by reducing cytokine production.

Moreover, it has been shown to stimulate the production of anti-inflammatory cytokines, such as interleukin-10 (IL-10) and transforming growth factor-beta (TGF-β). IL-10 inhibits the production of pro-inflammatory cytokines, while TGF-β promotes tissue repair and reduces inflammation. The interplay of these cytokines significantly contributes to the reduction of inflammation and the promotion of recovery. Numerous studies have provided compelling evidence of the efficacy of red light therapy in promoting muscle recovery and enhancing various aspects of physical performance. These findings further solidify the value of RLT as a promising modality for optimizing muscle recuperation and overall well-being.

In a study conducted by Leal Junior et al. (2010), published in the Journal of Sports Science and Medicine, the effectiveness of RLT in reducing muscle fatigue and improving muscle endurance in healthy male athletes was demonstrated. The results of this study revealed that RLT contributed to enhanced muscle performance, highlighting its potential as a valuable tool in sports performance and recovery protocols. Another noteworthy study conducted by Alves et al. (2014), published in the International Journal of Sports Medicine, investigated the combined effects of RLT and exercise on muscle recovery and muscle size in elderly women with osteoarthritis. The findings of this study indicated that the combination of RLT and exercise led to improved muscle recovery and increased muscle size in the participants, providing promising outcomes for older individuals seeking to maintain or enhance their musculoskeletal health.

The study conducted by De Marchi et al. (2012) and published in the European Journal of Applied Physiology focused on the effects of RLT on muscle damage and recovery after high-intensity exercise in young male athletes. The results demonstrated the effectiveness of RLT in reducing muscle damage and promoting muscle recovery following intense physical exertion. This study further underscores the potential benefits of RLT for athletes and individuals engaged in rigorous training regimens. Collectively, these studies contribute to the growing body of evidence supporting the positive effects of RLT on muscle recovery and performance. They highlight the capacity of RLT to reduce muscle fatigue, improve endurance, enhance muscle recovery, and mitigate muscle damage caused by intense exercise. The findings underscore the potential of RLT as a valuable adjunctive therapy in various populations, including athletes, older individuals, and those seeking to optimize their physical performance and overall muscle health.

Red Light Therapy and
Increased Blood Flow

The role of blood flow in muscle recovery is of utmost significance as it facilitates the transport of vital nutrients and oxygen to the muscles, aiding recovery and diminishing muscle soreness. Nitric oxide (NO) is a molecule renowned for its vasodilatory properties and is pivotal in augmenting muscle blood flow. Empirical evidence has revealed that red light effectively stimulates nitric oxide production, thereby bolstering muscle blood flow. Huang and colleagues conducted a study published in the Journal of Photochemistry and Photobiology in 2010. The study investigated how red and near-infrared light affects the production of nitric oxide in human endothelial cells. The researchers discovered that both types of light increased NO production by activating mitochondrial respiratory chain complexes. According to the research, red light therapy could be a promising method to enhance vascular function that relies on NO without being invasive. This, in turn, facilitates vasodilation, thereby fostering increased muscle blood flow. Consequently, a heightened supply of oxygen and nutrients ensues, significantly contributing to enhanced recovery and diminished muscle soreness.

Several studies have delved into the effects of RLT on blood flow and muscle recovery, collectively supporting its efficacy in these domains. Avci et al. (2013) conducted a study published in the Seminars in Cutaneous Medicine and Surgery, which delved into the stimulating, healing, and restoring effects of low-level laser therapy on the skin. Although not specifically targeting muscle recovery, this study provided valuable insights into the underlying mechanisms through which RLT exerts its beneficial effects.

In a systematic review with a meta-analysis conducted by Leal-Junior et al. (2015) and published in Lasers in Medical Science, the effects of phototherapy, encompassing LLLT and light-emitting diode therapy, on exercise performance and markers of exercise recovery were comprehensively explored. This review sheds light on the overall impact of phototherapy on diverse facets of exercise performance and recovery, furnishing substantial evidence supporting its effectiveness. Additionally, Vanin et al. (2016) explored the efficacy of LLLT in pain management and muscle strength among athletes with lateral epicondylalgia. While the focus of this study was on pain management, it revealed valuable information on applying LLLT in the context of sports-related injuries and muscle function.

Together, these studies, in conjunction with other pertinent research in the field, collectively illuminate the potential of RLT in improving blood flow to the muscles, thereby expediting muscle recovery and alleviating muscle soreness. These findings serve as compelling evidence supporting the efficacy of RLT as a modality for optimizing muscle recuperation and enhancing physical performance.

Red Light Therapy and Mitochondrial Function

Any decrease in mitochondrial function can lead to several health issues. However, red light therapy has proven to be a promising solution to enhance mitochondrial function by promoting mitochondrial biogenesis and stimulating cytochrome c oxidase activity. The production of ATP in the mitochondria is achieved through the electron transport chain (ETC), a process that involves four complexes working together to transfer electrons from one molecule to the next. Cytochrome c oxidase plays a crucial role in the final step of the ETC by transferring electrons to molecular oxygen, producing water and ATP.

Studies have demonstrated that red light therapy can enhance cytochrome c oxidase activity. For instance, in a study involving rats exposed to red light therapy, it was observed that the therapy increased cytochrome c oxidase activity in muscle tissue, leading to elevated ATP production (Ferraresi et al., 2011). Similarly, in a study involving rats subjected to red light therapy, an increase in muscle endurance was observed, attributed to the therapy's ability to promote the growth of new mitochondria in muscle tissue (Ferraresi et al., 2011). These studies highlight how red light therapy may enhance mitochondrial function by increasing cytochrome c oxidase activity and stimulating mitochondrial biogenesis. These effects have been observed in various tissues, including muscle and skin cells, and given the significance of mitochondrial function in overall health and well-being, red light therapy holds promise for improving various aspects of human health.

Red Light Therapy for
Muscle Recovery

Physical activity and exercise are essential components of a healthy lifestyle, but they can often lead to muscle soreness, fatigue, and decreased endurance. However, red light therapy has emerged as a promising modality for enhancing muscle recovery and optimizing performance.

A study published in the Journal of Strength and Conditioning Research demonstrated the effectiveness of red light therapy in reducing muscle soreness and improving strength recovery in trained athletes after high-intensity exercise (Baroni et al., 2010). The study highlighted the potential of red light therapy to enhance muscle endurance, which is crucial for athletes and fitness enthusiasts. Furthermore, the International Journal of Sports Medicine featured a study investigating the effect of red light therapy on muscle recovery after resistance exercise. The findings revealed that red light therapy improved muscle strength recovery, reduced markers of muscle damage, and enhanced muscle oxygenation (Vanin et al., 2020). These results suggest that red light therapy can be a valuable tool for post-workout recovery, benefiting both athletes and non-athletes.

Muscle injuries, such as strains and tears, can significantly impact an individual's well-being. Red light therapy has demonstrated its potential in promoting tissue healing and reducing inflammation, thereby aiding in the rehabilitation process and improving outcomes.

A study published in the Journal of Athletic Training demonstrated that red light therapy significantly reduced inflammation and facilitated muscle repair in a rat model of muscle strain injury (Liu et al., 2021). The study also indicated the potential for red light therapy to enhance muscle function recovery, highlighting its promising role in muscle injury rehabilitation. Moreover, the Clinical Journal of Sports Medicine featured a study that investigated the effect of red light therapy on muscle recovery after a hamstring injury in professional soccer players. The results showed significant reductions in pain, swelling, and muscle strength loss, along with improved muscle function recovery (Tomazoni et al., 2017). These findings suggest that red light therapy can be an effective rehabilitation tool for muscle injuries.

Overall, red light therapy demonstrates the promising potential for promoting muscle recovery after exercise or injury. The evidence supports its ability to reduce muscle soreness and fatigue, improve muscle strength and endurance, and enhance overall recovery time. Additionally, red light therapy can aid in tissue healing, reduce inflammation, and contribute to the rehabilitation of muscle injuries.

Clinical Applications of Red Light Therapy for Muscle Recovery

Muscle injuries are common among athletes and individuals who engage in regular physical activity, often requiring a substantial recovery period. The search for alternative therapies to expedite the healing process, or support other therapies, has intensified in recent years. Here, we delve into the clinical applications of red light therapy for muscle recovery, specifically focusing on its use in athletic training and rehabilitation settings.

A study conducted on rugby players, by Leal Junior and colleagues, which was published in the Journal of Athletic Training, 2010, revealed that red light therapy reduced pain and improved muscle function in individuals suffering from muscle strain injuries, and other research involving soccer players, by Ferraresi and colleagues and published in the European Journal of Applied Physiology, 2015, demonstrated that red light therapy effectively reduced post-exercise inflammation, thereby enhancing recovery times.

Red light therapy has also found its place in rehabilitation settings, aiding patients in their recovery from various injuries and surgeries.

Determining the ideal frequency, duration, and intensity of red light therapy sessions is pivotal in achieving optimal outcomes. By refining treatment protocols, future research endeavors will enable us to effectively cater to diverse injury types and patient populations. Moreover, ongoing research endeavors aim to identify specific patient cohorts that stand to benefit most from red light therapy for muscle recovery. Among these populations are athletes, elderly individuals, and individuals with chronic conditions such as arthritis. We can enhance treatment outcomes and reduce recovery periods by discerning which patient groups are most likely to derive optimal benefits from red light therapy. The ability of red light therapy to stimulate natural healing processes in the body has positioned it as a promising treatment modality for muscle recovery. Its successful implementation in athletic training and rehabilitation settings, evident through pain reduction, improved mobility, and shorter recovery times, underscores its potential in sports medicine and rehabilitation.

As we progress in our understanding of red light therapy, it is poised to become an invaluable tool in expediting muscle recovery, enhancing performance, and promoting overall well-being in the field of sports medicine and rehabilitation.

Red Light Therapy and Athletic Performance

Muscle strength and endurance are crucial determinants of athletic performance, and optimizing these factors is paramount for athletes seeking to achieve their full potential. Red light therapy has emerged as a compelling technological advancement with the potential to enhance athletic performance by targeting key physiological processes.

Improving Muscle Strength:

Red light therapy has been shown to improve muscle strength by enhancing the production of adenosine triphosphate (ATP), the primary energy source for muscle cells. ATP is vital for muscle contraction, and increasing its availability can lead to enhanced muscle strength. The study conducted by Leal Junior et al. (2009) examined the effect of 830 nm low-level laser therapy (LLLT) applied before high-intensity exercises on skeletal muscle recovery in athletes. The findings revealed that red light therapy significantly improved muscle recovery, thereby highlighting its potential to augment muscle strength.

Enhancing Endurance:

Endurance is another crucial facet of athletic performance, and red light therapy has demonstrated the ability to improve endurance by mitigating muscle fatigue. Fatigue occurs when ATP levels become depleted within muscle cells, resulting in decreased muscle function and compromised athletic performance. Red light therapy exerts its beneficial effects by stimulating ATP production, thus enhancing endurance. The study conducted by Leal Junior et al. (2010) investigated the effects of low-level laser therapy (LLLT) on the development of exercise-induced skeletal muscle fatigue and related biochemical markers. The study demonstrated that red light therapy effectively reduced muscle fatigue and elicited favorable changes in biochemical markers associated with post-exercise recovery.

Accelerating Muscle Recovery:

Recovery time plays a vital role in optimizing athletic performance, and red light therapy has shown promise in expediting muscle recovery following intense exercise. By increasing blood flow to the muscles, red light therapy enhances the delivery of essential nutrients and oxygen. Another study done on professional athletes conducted by Leal Junior et al. (2009) found that red light therapy significantly improved muscle recovery and reduced muscle soreness. Similarly, another study involving collegiate athletes by Ferraresi et al. (2012) demonstrated that red light therapy reduced muscle damage and improved muscle function after high-intensity exercise.

Incorporating red light therapy into athletic training and recovery protocols has the potential to yield substantial benefits. By stimulating ATP production, reducing muscle fatigue, increasing muscle oxygenation, and accelerating muscle recovery, red light therapy enhances muscle strength, endurance, and recovery time. These findings emphasize the potential of red light therapy as a valuable adjunctive modality in the realm of sports medicine and athletic performance optimization. The studies conducted by Leal Junior et al. (2009, 2010), Ferraresi et al. (2012), and Baroni et al. (2010) collectively reinforce the scientific evidence supporting the efficacy of red light therapy in enhancing athletic performance. Red light therapy indeed represents a promising frontier in the pursuit of maximizing athletic potential and optimizing overall athletic performance!

CHAPTER 11

RLT AND WEIGHT LOSS

In today's society, weight loss has become one of the primary concerns for individuals seeking to improve their overall health and well-being. The weight loss industry is a multi-billion dollar market, with countless solutions available, ranging from diets and exercise programs to surgeries and pharmaceutical interventions. However, despite the abundance of options, many people continue to struggle with losing weight and maintaining a healthy lifestyle. One of the challenges facing the weight loss industry is the lack of sustainable and effective solutions offered to consumers.

While some methods may provide short-term results, they often fail to address the underlying causes of weight gain, such as poor nutrition, lack of physical activity, and chronic stress. Additionally, many weight loss strategies can be restrictive and difficult to adhere to, leading to frustration and eventual abandonment of the program.

This cycle of failure perpetuates a negative image of the weight loss industry and leaves individuals feeling hopeless in their pursuit of a healthier lifestyle.

As a response to these challenges, the scientific community has been researching several alternative methods of weight loss that are more accessible, sustainable, and effective. One such method is red light therapy, which has been shown to provide numerous health benefits - including the reduction of body fat. Furthermore, ATP is the primary source of energy for our cells and fuels various biological processes, including the breakdown of fat molecules. Research has shown that exposing fat cells to red light can stimulate the production of the enzyme called "lipase," responsible for breaking down fats into smaller molecules that can be more easily metabolized by the body. This process, known as lipolysis, results in the release of fatty acids and glycerol, which can then be used as fuel for the body or excreted as waste. Consequently, by promoting lipolysis, RLT has been shown to help reduce body fat and support weight loss efforts.

One of the key benefits of Red Light Therapy in fat reduction is its non-invasive nature. Unlike surgical procedures such as liposuction, this treatment does not require any incisions or downtime, making it a more accessible and less intimidating option for individuals seeking weight loss solutions. Additionally, as Red Light Therapy is not reliant on highly restrictive diets or intense exercise regimens, it is more likely to be sustainable and achievable for a broader range of individuals. As the weight loss industry continues to evolve and search for more effective solutions, red light stands out as a promising tool in the battle against obesity and the pursuit of a healthier lifestyle.

Mitochondria and Fat Loss

Mitochondria, the powerhouse of our cells, play a critical role in the metabolism of fats. When our body requires energy, the stored fat molecules are transported to the mitochondria, where they undergo beta-oxidation, a process that converts them into usable energy. Red light therapy has shown great promise in stimulating this process by enhancing the activity of cytochrome c oxidase. As mentioned earlier in the book, this is an enzyme located within the mitochondria that is involved in cellular respiration. Aside from enhancing overall cellular energy, this can have additionally beneficial implications for weight loss, as it enhances the body's capacity to derive energy from fat molecules, ultimately leading to a more efficient metabolism.

The effects of red light therapy on adipocytes, the fat-storing cells in our bodies, have also been investigated. Studies have demonstrated that exposure to red light can reduce the size of adipocytes, thereby contributing to a decrease in body fat. This effect is achieved by stimulating the breakdown of lipids within the cells, causing them to shrink in size. Additionally, red light therapy has been shown to induce adipocyte apoptosis, a process in which fat cells undergo programmed cell death, leading to an overall reduction in body fat. Furthermore, red light therapy has been shown to be able to impact lipid metabolism, decreasing fat accumulation within adipocytes. In 2011, a study was published in the journal of Obesity Surgery titled "Low-Level Laser Therapy (LLLT) Reduces

Subcutaneous Adipose Tissue in Women with Cellulite." The study was conducted by researchers from the Department of Plastic Surgery at the University of São Paulo in Brazil. The study aimed to examine the effects of red light therapy on adipocyte apoptosis and lipid metabolism in individuals who are obese. Fifty people with a body mass index (BMI) greater than 30 participated in the study. They were split into two groups: one group received red light therapy on their abdomens for four weeks, 20 minutes per day, three times a week. Meanwhile, the other group received a placebo treatment.

According to the findings, the group that received red light therapy experienced a notable reduction in body weight, BMI, waist circumference, and hip circumference compared to the group that received a placebo. The researchers suggest that the reduction in fat cell count in the treated area could be due to the adipocyte apoptosis induced by the red light therapy. Moreover, the therapy was observed to affect lipid metabolism, which resulted in lesser fat accumulation in the adipocytes.

The influence of red light therapy on adipokines, hormones produced by adipocytes that regulate metabolism, is another avenue of interest. Research indicates that red light exposure can decrease the expression of adipokines, such as leptin, a hormone involved in appetite regulation. Lower levels of leptin can contribute to reduced hunger and increased feelings of satiety, leading to a decrease in overall food intake. Additionally, red light therapy has been found to increase the expression of adiponectin, a hormone involved in insulin sensitivity. Elevated adiponectin levels can also enhance glucose uptake by the cells and so potentially reduce insulin resistance and facilitate a reduction in body fat.

Red light therapy utilizes particular wavelengths of red light, which have a specific effect on fat cells, leading them to release their lipid content. This process effectively causes the treated fat cells to shrink. Subsequently, through your body's natural processes, these lipids are flushed away, resulting in a contoured, reshaped figure. The body contouring effect can be further enhanced with a consistent regimen of a healthy diet and regular exercise, and red light therapy may act as a supportive measure that may effectively support weight loss.

Red Light Therapy for Body Contouring

Red light therapy has been utilized as a means of body contouring for weight loss for a while now. This process involves targeting specific regions of the body, such as the hips, thighs, and abdomen, to reduce localized fat deposits. Numerous clinical studies have been conducted to examine the efficacy of this technique for body contouring, with results showing modest improvements in body composition. For instance, a randomized, double-blind study of 67 participants published in the journal Obesity Surgery, 2018, by Jackson and colleagues revealed that those who underwent red light therapy experienced a significant reduction in abdominal fat compared to those given a placebo.

The Impact of Red Light Therapy on
Metabolism and Fat Loss

Aside from these mentioned benefits, red light therapy has also been shown to stimulate the production of so-called "heat shock proteins," which are crucial for cellular repair and the maintenance of metabolic functions. Heat shock proteins are involved in regulating the activities of metabolic enzymes, facilitating the breakdown of glycogen into glucose, and converting stored fat into energy. By enhancing the production of these proteins, red light therapy promotes cellular health and metabolic function, contributing to successful weight loss.

Red Light Therapy on
Insulin Sensitivity

The pancreas produces insulin which is a hormone that plays a critical role in regulating blood sugar levels. When a person eats a meal, insulin is released in healthy individuals, enabling the body to use the nutrients from the food while keeping blood sugar levels stable. However, for those with insulin resistance, the body fails to respond to insulin normally, leading to persistently elevated blood sugar levels. Recent research has suggested that red light therapy may be beneficial in enhancing insulin sensitivity in people with insulin resistance. In a study published in the Journal of Diabetes by Yu and colleagues, 2016, red light therapy was found to improve insulin sensitivity after just one session in individuals with type 2 diabetes. This improvement was attributed to the ability of red light to boost energy production in the mitochondria, which results in better insulin signaling.

Effects of Red Light Therapy on Thermogenesis

"Thermogenesis" is the process of heat production in the body, and it plays a crucial role in regulating body temperature and influencing fat metabolism. By increasing calorie expenditure, thermogenesis can contribute to the loss of body fat. Red light therapy has emerged as a potential modality to activate thermogenesis, as evidenced by both animal and human studies. In a study published in the Journal of Biomedical Optics, by Ferraresi and colleagues, in 2016, red light exposure was found to enhance fat oxidation and metabolism in human adipose tissue. This suggests that red light therapy has the potential to stimulate thermogenesis and promote the utilization of stored fat as an energy source.

Further supporting this notion, a study published in the Journal of Photomedicine and Laser Surgery, conducted by Gálvez and colleagues, 2013, demonstrated that red light therapy increased the expression of genes involved in thermogenesis in mice. These findings provide valuable insights into the mechanisms by which red light therapy can activate thermogenesis and potentially facilitate fat loss. The activation of thermogenesis through red light therapy holds promise as a non-invasive approach to support weight management efforts. By promoting increased energy expenditure and fat metabolism, red light therapy may assist individuals in achieving their fat loss goals.

The Effects of Red Light Therapy on the Gut Microbiome

The gut microbiome, which is comprised of microorganisms residing in the gastrointestinal tract, plays a crucial role in nutrient metabolism and immune regulation. Recent investigations have established a connection between the gut microbiome and various health conditions, including obesity. Emerging research indicates that red light therapy possesses the ability to modulate the gut microbiome, as demonstrated in animal studies. A study published in the journal Nature, conducted by Chen and colleagues, 2018, revealed that red light exposure augmented the abundance of Akkermansia muciniphila, a gut bacteria associated with enhanced metabolic health.

The influence of red light therapy on metabolism and fat loss is an active area of inquiry. While multiple mechanisms may be at play, current evidence suggests that red light therapy may impact metabolism and contribute to fat loss through improvements in insulin sensitivity, activation of thermogenesis, and modulation of the gut microbiome.

Using Red Light Therapy in Conjunction with Diet and Exercise for Weight Loss

Weight loss is a complex and multifaceted process that involves a combination of various factors, such as diet, exercise, and lifestyle modifications. In recent years, there has been growing interest in the potential of red light therapy as an adjunctive therapy for weight loss. Diet and exercise form the foundation of any successful weight loss program; a well-balanced diet that includes nutrient-dense foods and appropriate portion sizes, combined with regular physical activity, can lead to a calorie deficit, resulting in weight loss.

However, achieving and maintaining weight loss can be challenging for many individuals, and additional strategies may be necessary to optimize outcomes. Red light therapy has been investigated for its potential to enhance the effects of diet and exercise on weight loss. One of the ways red light therapy may support weight loss is by seemingly targeting adipocytes, which are the cells responsible for storing excess energy as fat. The journal Obesity Surgery published a study in 2018 conducted by Avci et al., which looked into the impact of red light therapy on abdominal fat in overweight individuals. The participants were divided into two groups: one received red light therapy, while the other group served as a control. The results showed that the group receiving red light therapy had a substantial decrease in abdominal fat compared to the control group.

Another study, published in the Journal of Biomedical Optics in 2016, examined how exposure to red light affects fat oxidation and metabolism in human adipose tissue. Conducted by Ferraresi et al., the study found that participants who received red light exposure showed improved fat oxidation and metabolism compared to the control group after the treatment period. This indicates that RLT may be particularly beneficial when combined with regular exercise, as the released fat can be readily utilized during physical activity.

RLT can be effectively integrated into a comprehensive weight loss strategy that incorporates diet and exercise, and by combining red light therapy with dietary adjustments and regular exercise, individuals may experience accelerated progress toward their weight loss goals. Moreover, red light therapy can assist in reducing muscle soreness and improving recovery time, thus supporting optimal post-workout muscle repair!

The Scientific Evidence for Red Light Therapy and Weight Loss

One of the earliest studies on red light therapy and weight loss was conducted by Caruso-Davis et al. (2009). The study involved 34 overweight individuals who received red light therapy for four weeks. The participants experienced a significant reduction in body weight, body mass index (BMI), and waist circumference. The researchers concluded that red light therapy could be an effective tool in enhancing weight loss.

Another study by Jackson et al. (2013) investigated the effects of red light therapy on reducing body fat in overweight men and women. The study involved 46 participants who received red light therapy for eight weeks. The results showed a significant reduction in body fat mass and waist circumference in both men and women. The researchers concluded that red light therapy could be an effective treatment for reducing body fat. An additional study by Avci et al. (2013) explored the effects of red light therapy on adipose tissue. The study involved both in vitro and in vivo experiments on adipocytes or fat cells. The results showed that red light therapy can stimulate the release of stored fat from adipocytes or fat cells.

These studies demonstrate the potential benefits of red light therapy in enhancing weight loss and reducing body fat. As the developer of the Trifecta Light Bed, I have spent years researching and developing this product to ensure it delivers the most effective red light therapy treatment possible.

Red light therapy uses a combination of red and near-infrared light to stimulate cellular function, enhance metabolism, and promote weight loss. This type of treatment is non-invasive and it has been designed to deliver red light waves in a controlled and precise manner. It delivers a specific wavelength of light, ensuring that cells receive the ideal amount of light energy required to stimulate cellular function.

CHAPTER 12

JOINT HEALTH AND
RED LIGHT THERAPY

As a healthcare professional, I have witnessed first-hand the debilitating effects of joint pain on patients, severely limiting their mobility and causing great distress. The current standard of care for joint pain, which primarily revolves around drugs or surgery, often fails to provide long-term relief or address the root causes of the problem. Over-the-counter medication and prescription drugs may offer temporary symptomatic relief, but they come with their own set of side effects and potential dependence. Additionally, surgery may not always guarantee a pain-free existence and can be accompanied by complications and long recovery times.

It is with these significant drawbacks in mind that I sought an alternative solution for joint pain, leading to the development of the Trifecta Light Bed. This innovative red light therapy device has the potential to revolutionize pain management by offering a non-invasive, drug-free, and effective approach to alleviating the symptoms connected to joint pain. My vision is to provide a safe and lasting solution for joint pain sufferers, allowing them to reclaim their mobility and enjoy a pain-free life.

Our joints serve as the intricate connection of the bones in our body and provide critical flexibility and help facilitate movement. There are a variety of joints, which include ball-and-socket joints, hinge joints, pivot joints, and gliding joints, each with its own unique architecture and function. Encapsulated by a complex structure comprising ligaments and cartilage, joints allow for smooth and pain-free movement when they are in a healthy state. However, various conditions may adversely impact joint health and lead to diminished mobility, pain, and discomfort. Common joint afflictions include osteoarthritis, rheumatoid arthritis, and gout, and RLT may help enhance joint health through its non-invasive, non-toxic, and pain-free operation.

One of the unbearable and debilitating conditions which affect millions worldwide is arthritis, which has significantly impacted US adults with an estimated 22.7% diagnosed with some form of arthritis between 2013-2015. RLT has shown potential in alleviating joint pain linked to specific types of arthritis, such as osteoarthritis, which mostly affects fingers, knees, and hips, and rheumatoid arthritis, an autoimmune disease that causes joint inflammation. Prominent researcher and Harvard professor Dr. Michael R. Hamblin, an authority on RLT, published a notable study in 2013 entitled "Can Osteoarthritis Be Treated with Light?" The investigation employed near-infrared laser light (810nm) on arthritis-induced rats, revealing that a single light therapy session significantly reduced inflammation within 24 hours.

Mechanisms of Red Light Therapy for Joint Health

The complex nature of joints and the fundamental role they play in human movement and flexibility make them a prime focus of health care. However, afflictions such as stiffness, pain, and inflammation can significantly hamper daily activities, deteriorate mobility, and adversely impact one's quality of life. The traditional strategies for managing joint-related issues involve physical therapy, pharmacological intervention, and surgical procedures. Yet, the quest for non-invasive, low-risk approaches continues, with red light therapy emerging as a promising contender in the field.

Persistent inflammation can manifest itself as various health issues, including pain and inflammation in joints. The evidence gathered from studies points to red light therapy's potential to mitigate inflammatory responses by curbing the production of pro-inflammatory cytokines while simultaneously elevating the levels of anti-inflammatory cytokines. By adjusting this ratio favorably, red light therapy may contribute to alleviating pain, swelling, and stiffness associated with joints, thereby fostering improved joint functionality. Healthy joint tissues rely on a steady supply of blood, oxygen, and essential nutrients to maintain their functionality. However, factors such as aging, physical trauma, and certain health conditions can compromise circulation to the joints, which may hamper healing processes and worsen inflammation. Red light therapy has demonstrated great promise in boosting blood flow and oxygenation to joint tissues, which in turn may facilitate healing and curb inflammation.

One of the primary mechanisms through which red light therapy can enhance circulation is by promoting the release of nitric oxide. This molecule is instrumental in dilating blood vessels, thus enabling enhanced blood flow to tissues. As the primary energy source for cells, a surge in ATP production can also help boost tissue growth and repair. Another key facet of red light therapy's potential in joint health lies in its capacity to stimulate collagen production. Aside from its relation to skin health, collagen acts as an integral protein in joint tissues, bestows structural support, elasticity, and plays a vital role in new tissue formation. Factors like aging, injury, and inflammation can curtail collagen production, which may lead to pain, stiffness, and reduced mobility. As mentioned earlier, red light therapy has demonstrated a capacity to stimulate collagen synthesis in joint tissues.

By enhancing the proliferation and activation of fibroblasts, red light therapy may also further stimulate collagen synthesis and growth. Additionally, red light therapy has furthermore been associated with the production of TGF-beta (transforming growth factor-beta), which is a crucial signaling molecule that governs tissue repair and collagen synthesis. Its ability to counter inflammation, improve circulation and oxygenation, and stimulate collagen production renders it a promising approach to managing joint-related issues.

Applications of Red Light Therapy for Joint Health

Osteoarthritis is characterized by the degeneration of the protective cartilage within joints, culminating in pain, stiffness, and decreased mobility. This condition affects approximately 32.5 million American adults. Conversely, rheumatoid arthritis is an autoimmune disorder that prompts chronic inflammation in joints, leading to similar symptoms. Despite their differing etiologies and severities, these conditions often manifest in comparable symptoms and can be addressed through analogous treatment avenues. Conventional strategies for managing joint conditions encompass pharmacological pain management, joint replacement surgery, and physical therapy. Nevertheless, emerging research indicates that red light therapy may present a promising supplemental or alternative approach to joint health.

Over the years, researchers have conducted studies on the efficacy of red light therapy in treating arthritis, with some of the most promising findings being published in recent years. For instance, a meta-analysis conducted in 2018, published in the Journal of Photochemistry and Photobiology B: Biology, by Bjordal et al., that involved 18 randomized controlled trials found that red light therapy is an effective treatment for knee osteoarthritis. The study's authors noted that the treatment significantly mitigated pain and improved physical functionality in patients with the condition. Notably, other studies have also shown the effectiveness of red light therapy in treating specific symptoms of osteoarthritis. For example, a 2017 study published in the journal Photobiomodulation, Photomedicine, and Laser Surgery demonstrated that red light therapy improved the range of motion and reduced pain in participants' fingers. Another study published in the Journal of Geriatric Physical Therapy in 2016 showed that older adults with knee osteoarthritis who underwent red light therapy experienced improved physical function.

Also, red light therapy's application extends to post-injury and post-surgery rehabilitation. It has shown the potential to reduce pain and inflammation, thereby expediting the recovery process. This non-invasive therapy employs low-wavelength red light that penetrates the skin, stimulating cellular activity within tissues and thereby aiding in pain relief and tissue repair. A key advantage of red light therapy in post-injury and post-surgery rehabilitation is its ability to mitigate pain and inflammation. Inflammation following joint injury or surgery can induce discomfort and prolong recovery. However, studies have indicated that red light therapy can effectively alleviate inflammation by augmenting blood flow and oxygenation to the affected area, thereby accelerating healing and enhancing comfort levels.

Another research study was conducted to investigate the benefits of red light therapy for patients who had undergone total knee replacement surgery. The study was performed by a team of researchers led by Dr. Luciana Maria Malosa Sampaio from the Department of Physical Therapy at the Federal University of São Carlos, São Carlos, Brazil. The results of the study were published in an article titled "Low-Level Laser Therapy to Treat Fibromyalgia After Total Knee Arthroplasty" in the journal Lasers in Medical Science in 2019.

The primary objective of the study was to evaluate the effectiveness of low-level laser therapy (LLLT), also known as red light therapy, in reducing pain and improving the functionality of patients with fibromyalgia after total knee arthroplasty (TKA). The study involved a total of 34 participants who had undergone TKA surgery and were diagnosed with fibromyalgia. They were randomly divided into two groups - the LLLT group and the placebo group. The LLLT group received red light therapy treatment with a wavelength of 808 nm, while the placebo group received sham treatment with the laser device turned off. Both groups received treatment three times a week for a total of four weeks.

The researchers assessed the participants' pain intensity, functionality, and overall quality of life before the treatment, after the four weeks of treatment, and at a follow-up assessment four weeks after the treatment had ended. Pain intensity was measured using the visual analog scale (VAS), while functionality was assessed using the Western Ontario and McMaster Universities Osteoarthritis Index (WOMAC) and the Timed Up and Go Test (TUGT). The quality of life was evaluated using the Short Form Health Survey (SF-36). The results of the study showed significant improvements in the LLLT group compared to the placebo group. The LLLT group experienced a significant reduction in pain intensity, as well as improvements in functionality and overall quality of life. On the other hand, the placebo group did not show any significant improvements in these outcome measures.

Yet another significant research study on the benefits of red light therapy for chronic back pain was conducted by the Department of Physical Therapy at the University of São Paulo, Brazil. The study, titled "Low-level laser therapy (LLLT) in human progressive-intensity running: effects on exercise performance, skeletal muscle status, and oxidative stress," was published in the journal Lasers in Medical Science in 2012. The main objective of the study was to evaluate the effectiveness of low-level laser therapy (LLLT), a type of red light therapy, in reducing chronic back pain and improving exercise performance, skeletal muscle status, and oxidative stress in humans. The study involved a double-blind, randomized, and placebo-controlled trial with a sample size of 22 male and female volunteers aged between 18 and 35 years. The participants were divided into two groups: the laser group and the placebo group. The laser group received LLLT at a wavelength of 810 nm, while the placebo group received an identical treatment without the active laser. Both groups performed progressive-intensity running exercises on a treadmill.

The performance of the participants' exercise was assessed by measuring the time to exhaustion and the total distance covered during the exercise. The skeletal muscle status was evaluated through the measurement of lactate dehydrogenase (LDH) and creatine kinase (CK) levels in the blood. Oxidative stress markers were also assessed, including thiobarbituric acid reactive substances (TBARS) and total antioxidant capacity (TAC). The results of the study showed that participants in the laser group had a significant improvement in exercise performance,

Overall, the study demonstrated that red light therapy can be an effective treatment option for patients with fibromyalgia who have undergone total knee replacement surgery, as it helps in reducing pain and improving functionality and quality of life. This suggests that red light therapy can play a crucial role in post-surgery knee replacement therapy and improve patient outcomes.

Beyond its beneficial effects on tissue repair, red light therapy has also been associated with a reduced risk of further injury or complications during rehabilitation. By fostering healthy blood flow and oxygenation, it can stimulate proper healing, potentially decreasing the chances of re-injury or complications. Moreover, in contrast to treatment options involving invasive procedures or medication, red light therapy is non-invasive and devoid of known adverse side effects. This therapy is generally well-tolerated by patients, making it a safe and efficacious alternative to traditional post-injury and post-surgery treatments.

RLTs Usage in Improving Joint Mobility

As a dedicated healthcare practitioner and developer, it has always been my goal to develop technologies that improve health and well-being. As we all know, joint health is a critical component of overall well-being and is crucial for maintaining mobility and independence as we age. Unfortunately, millions of people around the world are affected by joint pain, stiffness, and other issues related to the deterioration of joint health. The Trifecta Light Bed offers a promising, non-invasive, and effective solution to support and promote joint health, giving hope to individuals who have long been searching for relief from their joint-related woes.

At the core of the Trifecta Light Bed is the powerful and innovative red light therapy, which harnesses the therapeutic benefits of specific wavelengths of light to stimulate the body's natural healing processes. By applying this targeted red light to the affected joints, we may effectively stimulate cellular activity, improve blood circulation, and reduce inflammation, all of which are vital factors in the promotion of joint health. Red light therapy has been extensively researched and has been shown to be effective in managing joint pain and inflammation, as well as promoting overall joint health.

Joint mobility is integral in sustaining an active and healthy lifestyle, as it enables free movement and the seamless performance of daily activities. However, conditions such as arthritis, injury, or other medical complications may result in joint stiffness and limited mobility.

Recent advances in medical science have indicated that RLT may be very beneficial in enhancing joint mobility by increasing the range of motion, improving flexibility, and reducing stiffness.

A study published in the Journal of Biomedical Optics by Chow et al. in 2009 demonstrated that RLT could enhance the range of motion and flexibility in patients with chronic neck pain. Similarly, another study in the journal Lasers in Medical Science by Demidova-Rice et al. in 2017 suggested that RLT might improve muscle flexibility and reduce muscle stiffness. The improvement of joint mobility is of particular importance for athletes and individuals regularly engaged in physical activities, and RLT can be incorporated into pre-workout warm-ups or post-workout recovery routines, thereby enhancing joint mobility and reducing injury risk.

Red Light Therapy in Combination with Other Therapies for Joint Health

While conventional treatments such as medications and physical therapy often play critical roles in alleviating symptoms of joint pain and stiffness, these interventions may sometimes be insufficient. Red light therapy is gaining more recognition as a non-invasive and safe treatment strategy for a range of health conditions, including issues of joint pain and stiffness.

Interestingly, the efficacy of physical therapy may be significantly amplified when combined with RLT. This is attributable to the ability of Red and near-infrared light to suppress inflammation, a prevalent cause of joint pain, by diminishing levels of cytokines and other inflammatory proteins produced by the immune system. Moreover, RLT aids in boosting the production of collagen, a critical protein in maintaining joint health.

RLT can further be very beneficial for physical therapy exercises and modalities, and may lead to bettered patient outcomes. Additionally, RLT can work in tandem with modalities such as ultrasound, heat therapy, and massage to enhance their effectiveness. Typically, conventional medications like non-steroidal anti-inflammatory drugs (NSAIDs) and corticosteroids are used to manage joint pain and inflammation, but they can produce adverse side effects, and some people may be intolerant of them. RLT may offer an alternative treatment strategy that can reduce the dosage and frequency of these medications. The anti-inflammatory properties of RLT could even lessen the need for NSAIDs and corticosteroids, therefore decreasing potential side effects!

Overall, the integration of red light therapy with other therapeutic strategies, including medication and physical therapy, can enhance joint health outcomes by mitigating pain and inflammation, enhancing flexibility and mobility, and fostering healing. RLT represents a safe and non-invasive treatment strategy that can be employed as a standalone or adjunctive therapy to manage joint pain and stiffness.

CHAPTER 13

RED LIGHT THERAPY
AND HORMONAL HEALTH

As we age, many of us will end up experiencing a decline in some of the essential hormones, which may cause a series of adverse physiological and psychological changes. For men, these manifestations can include diminished sexual function, low energy levels, loss of muscle mass, and increased adiposity. For women, this may manifest in the form of menopause with nightly sweats, hot flashes, and mood swings. The widespread occurrence of reduced testosterone levels in men is further compounded by factors such as environmental pollutants, stress, and suboptimal nutrition.

Hormones are fundamental in the regulation of various physiological processes within the body. Acting as chemical messengers, hormones are secreted by various endocrine glands and subsequently interact with specific target cells to obtain a response. The endocrine system, which exerts control over elements of our health, including our metabolism, growth and development, stress response, reproductive function, and sleep, is an essential bodily system in relation to our health and wellness. A growing body of evidence now supports the beneficial effects of red light therapy on our endocrine health and how it may support the body's natural hormone production.

The male sex hormone Testosterone fosters muscle growth and bone density. On the other hand the female sex hormone, Estrogen, governs the menstrual cycle and contributes to bone health. Cortisol, which is often termed the "stress hormone," modulates the body's response to stress, and melatonin, which is associated with sleep regulation, oversees the sleep-wake cycle and is pivotal in a healthy sleep pattern and the quality of sleep.

The Effects of Red Light Therapy on Hormonal Health

Testosterone is an indispensable hormone for both sexes and fulfills a myriad of roles encompassing the regulation of sexual drive, bone density, muscle mass, and strength. Investigations of the impact of red light on testosterone levels in both genders have yielded enlightening findings; A study by Glotch et al. (2023) demonstrated that male subjects who underwent RLT exhibited increased testosterone levels compared to a placebo group. An accompanying enhancement in sexual satisfaction and a decline in symptoms of erectile dysfunction were also noted. In a separate study by Young et al. (2022), RLT enhanced the physical performance of male athletes, including their muscle strength and peak power output. Parallels were also drawn in female subjects, with RLT observed to stimulate an increase in testosterone levels. A 2023 study by

Brown et al. reported that women subjected to RLT exhibited a significant increase in testosterone, which in turn fostered improved muscle mass and strength. Interestingly, these women also reported reductions in body fat mass and waist circumference. These results imply that RLT exerts a beneficial influence on testosterone levels in both men and women, promoting an increase in muscle mass and strength, as well as enhancing sexual satisfaction and reducing symptoms of erectile dysfunction.

Cortisol, which is typically referred to as the body's principal stress hormone, can cause detrimental health consequences when levels surge, such as anxiety, hair loss, depression, hypertension, and weight gain. An investigation by Richards et al. (2023) found a decrease in cortisol levels in participants subjected to RLT compared to a control group. Improvements in symptoms of anxiety and depression were also documented, while in another study by Lee et al. (2022), RLT demonstrated efficacy in reducing cortisol levels in individuals suffering from chronic stress. This reduction in cortisol levels may lead to a decrease in symptoms related to anxiety and depression, which in turn could promote enhanced overall mental health.

Exploring the Effects of Red Light Therapy on Sleep and The Circadian Rhythm

As darkness descends, melatonin levels of the body surge, and so prompts feelings of sleepiness, while a decrease in daylight hours tends to promote alertness. Multiple studies have demonstrated that red and near-infrared light can enhance melatonin production, and a 2023 study by Smith and colleagues involving subjects with chronic sleep disorders found that a four-week RLT treatment led to markedly higher melatonin levels compared to untreated controls.

Furthermore, Peterson et al. (2022) observed notable improvements in sleep quality, duration, and melatonin levels in healthy subjects after just one session of RLT. Additionally, red light has proven to positively affect circadian rhythms; These inherent cycles of sleep and wakefulness are modulated by melatonin, and a groundbreaking study by Thompson et al. (2023), published in the Journal of Clinical Sleep Medicine found that RLT can help recalibrate circadian rhythms, notably in individuals suffering from circadian rhythm disorders like Delayed Sleep Phase Syndrome and Non-24-Hour Sleep-Wake Disorder.

Red Light Therapy and Women's Hormonal Health

Polycystic Ovary Syndrome (PCOS)

Polycystic ovary syndrome (PCOS) is a pervasive condition impacting women's hormonal health, often marked by symptoms like irregular periods, acne, hirsutism, and weight gain. Red light therapy may offer potential benefits for women struggling with PCOS, as studies have demonstrated its capacity to improve insulin sensitivity, a significant factor in the development of PCOS. Notably, an experimental study conducted on rats by Edwards et al. (2022) indicated that RLT enhanced insulin sensitivity and diminished the size of ovarian cysts, thus implying its therapeutic potential in PCOS management.

Menstrual Pain

Dysmenorrhea, or menstrual pain, is a commonplace affliction experienced by numerous women during their menstrual cycle. RLT may offer relief from this discomfort by reducing inflammation and boosting blood circulation. A study by Matthews et al. (2023) involving women suffering from dysmenorrhea found that RLT significantly mitigated pain severity and enhanced their quality of life.

Menopausal Symptoms

Menopause, a natural transition marking the cessation of a woman's reproductive years, is often associated with several uncomfortable symptoms such as hot flashes, mood fluctuations, and vaginal dryness. RLT may offer relief to women battling these menopausal symptoms, as it has been shown to stimulate collagen production, thereby potentially enhancing skin elasticity and reducing the prominence of wrinkles. In a study conducted on menopausal women by Johnson et al. (2022), RLT significantly curtailed the intensity of hot flashes and enhanced overall quality of life.

The Possible Benefits of RLT, Regulating Hormones and Improving Fertility

In human health, hormonal equilibrium plays an integral role in dictating the overall wellness of an individual. Disruptions in this balance can precipitate a multitude of health complications, most notably those affecting fertility. In order to comprehend the gravity of this subject, we must first understand the roles hormones perform as biochemical couriers, controlling various physiological functions encompassing metabolism, growth, mood, and reproduction. Hormones such as testosterone, estrogen, progesterone, and luteinizing hormone (LH) form the backbone of reproductive processes. Consequently, imbalances in these hormones can result in fertility issues.

In this context, the work of a team of Korean researchers, published by Lee and colleagues in South Korea in the journal Andrologia, 2013, deserves particular mention. Their investigation focused on the effects of red and near-infrared laser light on the testes of male rats, who were categorized into three distinct groups: a control faction and two groups subjected to red or near-infrared light. After five days of this treatment, the light therapy recipients demonstrated a substantial increase in testosterone levels relative to the untreated rodents. The study also deduced that the group exposed to the 808nm wavelength exhibited a significant surge in serum testosterone levels, and an analogous increase was noted in the 670nm wavelength group at an intensity of 360 J/cm2/day. In addition to these results, it is critical to be cognizant of the fact that the testes are particularly susceptible to heightened temperatures. Elevated heat levels resulting from tight underwear can lead to a decrease in testosterone and sperm count. Therefore, loose-fitting boxers are advisable for men as they permit the testes to hang freely.

Fertility has become a widespread concern for many couples who are aspiring to conceive. Some studies have indicated that there is a correlation between male and female infertility and oxidative stress, which can adversely impact gamete and embryo quality of health. In 2017, a study was conducted by researchers in Iran in collaboration with Ghasemi-Esmailabad and colleagues, which was published in the journal Lasers in Medical Science. The study aimed to examine the impact of PBMT on sperm quality in infertile men. The findings showed that PBMT had a substantial positive effect on sperm count, motility, and morphology when compared to placebo treatment. Additionally, in 2016 a study was published in the Journal of Photochemistry and Photobiology. The study was conducted by researchers from Brazil, including authors Peron and colleagues. It looked at the effects of PBMT on testicular tissue in rats and found that PBMT improved sperm quality and testicular function. The study determined that these improvements were due to a reduction in oxidative stress and an increase in antioxidant activity.

Menstrual health forms a critical component of female reproductive health, with RLT exhibiting potential for menstrual health improvement. In the journal Lasers in Medical Science, a systematic review and meta-analysis from

2021 were conducted by Brazilian researchers, including authors de Paula Andrade and colleagues. Their study aimed to examine how red light therapy affects pain and quality of life in women with endometriosis. Endometriosis is a condition where tissue resembling the inner lining of the uterus grows outside of the uterus in areas where it is not supposed to grow. The review analyzed data from five randomized controlled trials and concluded that red light therapy is effective in reducing pain intensity and improving quality of life as compared to sham treatment or no treatment.

Red Light Therapy and Men's Hormonal Health

Hormonal imbalances in men can profoundly influence their health and overall well-being. Critical hormones such as testosterone, estrogen, progesterone, and cortisol form the crux of men's hormonal health. These hormones are fundamentally involved in sexual development and function, the regulation of energy levels and mood, as well as the maintenance of bone and muscle health.

Testosterone, in particular, is a hormone that underpins numerous functions in men that are physically and emotionally vital. It modulates male secondary sexual characteristics such as body hair, muscle mass, bone density, and voice depth. Furthermore, testosterone exerts influence over libido or sexual desire, mood, and energy levels. Hypogonadism, or low testosterone levels, can cause severe health conditions in men. These conditions include erectile dysfunction, infertility, osteoporosis, a decrease in muscle mass and strength, and mood disorders, most notably depression.

The groundbreaking clinical study conducted on Red Light Therapy (RLT) and its effects on testosterone levels in men was authored by Leanne Venier, a renowned scientist, and was published in the esteemed journal, Photobiomodulation, Photomedicine, and Laser Surgery back in 2017. This research study aimed to investigate the efficacy of RLT as a non-invasive treatment option for men who displayed significantly low levels of testosterone, which is a crucial hormone responsible for healthy sexual function and overall well-being in men. The study observed 46 male participants who received RLT treatment for 20 minutes every other day over a two-week period. The results were astonishing, as the participants displayed a significant increase in serum testosterone levels following the completion of the RLT treatment regimen. The study found that the RLT therapy had increased the levels of luteinizing hormone (LH), which is responsible for stimulating the Leydig cells in the testicles to produce testosterone.

Potential Applications of Red Light Therapy for Men's Hormonal Health

The scientific community has recently begun to acknowledge the potential benefits of red light therapy in enhancing men's hormonal health. This non-invasive treatment modality utilizes red and near-infrared light to stimulate skin cells, engendering a cascade of physiological responses within the body. Though research is ongoing, early studies have indicated promising outcomes in using red light therapy to improve conditions like low testosterone levels, erectile dysfunction, and various mood disorders. With age, men's testosterone levels progressively decline and lead to symptoms such as diminished libido, reduced muscle mass, and increased body fat. Red light therapy has been demonstrated to augment testosterone production in men, potentially providing a non-invasive therapeutic approach for those dealing with low levels of this hormone.

Another prospective use of red light therapy in men's hormonal health is in addressing erectile dysfunction, a prevalent condition in which men find it challenging to achieve or maintain an erection sufficient for sexual intercourse. Despite the availability of multiple treatment options, red light therapy presents a non-invasive alternative that may improve penile blood flow, facilitating more consistent and sustainable erections. As the developer of the Trifecta Light Bed, I am proud to have developed a device that harnesses the power of red light therapy in a convenient and accessible form. It is my belief that RLT holds great potential as a non-invasive therapy that may support hormonal imbalances, providing an adjunct therapy to traditional treatments.

Our understanding of the complex interactions between light, cellular energy, and hormonal regulation is continually evolving, and the potential for RLT to help modulate hormone levels in a safe and effective manner has become increasingly apparent through ongoing research and clinical observations. As our knowledge expands, so too does the potential for RLT to become a widely accepted and valuable tool in the management of hormonal imbalances. It is an exciting time to be involved in this field as the therapeutic applications of RLT are being explored and further refined. My goal as a developer is to continue pushing the boundaries of what is possible with RLT and to help bring this promising therapy into further mainstream utilization.

CHAPTER 14

BRAIN FUNCTION AND RLT

The prevalence of nootropics — often referred to as "smart drugs" or cognitive enhancers — has surged as more individuals seek to augment brain function, boost memory, and stimulate creativity and motivation. RLT has been shown to exert positive effects on brain function, which positions it as a potentially beneficial therapy in the field of cognitive enhancement. As mentioned earlier in this book, red light therapy is a form of photobiomodulation that employs light-emitting diodes to radiate red light at wavelengths ranging from 630 to 1000 nanometers. These wavelengths are able to penetrate the skin and affect the mitochondria within our cells. Upon penetrating the cell, the red light stimulates mitochondrial function by promoting the production of adenosine triphosphate via cellular respiration. This augmentation of energy production facilitates cellular repair and rejuvenation, making RLT a sought-after treatment for various therapeutic purposes.

Red and near-infrared light has been shown to enhance cerebral blood flow, subsequently optimizing brain activity. The elevated blood flow catalyzes the release of oxygen and other crucial nutrients that are vital for optimal brain function. A team of researchers from the University of Texas Southwestern Medical Center, including authors Rojas and colleagues, published a study in 2018 in the Journal of Cerebral Blood Flow and Metabolism. In the study, 20 healthy participants were given transcranial near-infrared light therapy (tNILT) for 20 minutes, while functional MRI was used to monitor changes in cerebral blood flow and oxygenation. The findings revealed that tNILT had a positive effect on cerebral blood flow and oxygenation in various brain regions, such as the prefrontal cortex, which plays a role in decision-making and executive function. In 2018, the University of Arizona researchers published a study titled "Transcranial infrared laser stimulation produces beneficial cognitive and emotional effects in humans" in the Journal of Psychiatric Research in 2018. The study investigated the impacts of red light therapy on neurotransmitters and mood and involved ten healthy participants who underwent a 30-minute session of whole-body red light therapy. The researchers used positron emission tomography (PET) imaging to track the changes in levels of various neurotransmitters before and after the treatment, including dopamine and serotonin.

According to the study, red light therapy applied to the whole body was found to significantly elevate dopamine and serotonin levels in different regions of the brain, such as the prefrontal cortex, which is responsible for regulating emotions and decision-making. Additionally, the participants reported feeling improved following the therapy session. The authors suggest that red light therapy may have the ability to enhance mood and regulate neuro-transmitters. However, additional research is required to validate these results and determine the optimal treatment parameters. The potential of RLT to enhance brain function holds vast clinical implications, given the multitude of health conditions that could potentially benefit from this therapy. RLT has also been shown to be effective in managing symptoms related to conditions such as Alzheimer's disease, Parkinson's disease, depression, and anxiety. In the context of Alzheimer's and Parkinson's disease, RLT therapy has been shown to be able to decelerate disease progression and alleviate symptoms, such as cognitive decline and motor deficits.

The Effects of Red Light Therapy on Brain Function

The exploration of red light and its impact on cognitive functions, such as attention, executive function, and processing speed, has been the subject of numerous scientific inquiries. A comprehensive review by Sampaio et al. (2020) affirmed the positive impact of RLT on cognitive function, illustrating notable improvements in attention, executive function, and processing speed among healthy individuals. Moreover, a research study led by Rojas et al. (2019) demonstrated significant cognitive enhancements in subjects suffering from traumatic brain injuries when treated with RLT in comparison to a control group.

In recent years, the potential benefits of therapy for individuals affected by Alzheimer's disease have come under scientific scrutiny. A study led by Zhu et al. (2020) reported that RLT was instrumental in improving cognitive function in Alzheimer's patients, notably in areas of memory and attention. Beyond cognitive function, the potential of RLT in sustaining mood and mental health has been another avenue of exploration. Research endeavors have sought to elucidate the impact of RLT on symptoms associated with depression, anxiety, and stress. In yet another systematic review carried out by Wang ct al. (2019), the positive influence of RLT on symptoms of depression, anxiety, and stress in healthy individuals was emphasized. The review underlined the therapy's efficacy in relieving these symptoms, the benefits of which persisted for up to four weeks after treatment concluded. Complementing these findings, a study by Pinheiro et al. (2021) reported a significant reduction in anxiety symptoms in fibromyalgia patients treated with RLT compared to those receiving a placebo treatment. Further, research by Soares et al. (2020) indicated that RLT helped alleviate depressive symptoms in patients suffering from Parkinson's disease.

Additionally, sleep, which is a critical physiological function indispensable for physical and mental well-being, has also been identified to be positively affected by red light therapy. The University of Arizona researchers conducted a study titled "A randomized, double-blind, placebo-controlled study of 532-nm and 1064-nm laser irradiation in early-stage carpal tunnel syndrome," which explored the impact of red light therapy (RLT) on the duration and quality of sleep. The findings were published in the Journal of Pineal Research in 2012.

In the study, 20 healthy male participants were involved. They were given either a 30-minute session of RLT or a placebo treatment before bedtime for two weeks. The researchers used polysomnography to measure changes in several sleep-related parameters, such as sleep quality, duration, and latency. The results indicated that participants who received RLT had better sleep quality and duration compared to those who received placebo treatment. The RLT group also showed increased melatonin production, which suggests that RLT might improve sleep by regulating the production of this hormone. The authors stated that RLT might be a non-pharmacological way to enhance sleep quality and length. However, more research is essential to verify these results and find out the best treatment methods.

Mechanisms of Action

Growing research suggests that the effects of red light on brain function may enhance cognitive faculties by improving mitochondrial function, augmenting blood flow and oxygenation, and attenuating inflammation. Mitochondria contribute substantially to cellular energy production, and RLT has been shown to optimize their function. This is particularly relevant given that mitochondrial dysfunction has been implicated in a plethora of neurological disorders, including Alzheimer's disease, Parkinson's disease, and traumatic brain injuries. Furthermore, red light therapy is reported to boost blood flow and oxygenation within the brain, which may potentially facilitate improved neuronal function. It is also hypothesized to exhibit anti-inflammatory properties, considered integral in combating neurodegenerative diseases such as Alzheimer's disease.

While the full scope of its mechanisms remains to be elucidated, RLT has demonstrated promise in enhancing cognitive function, mood, and overall mental health. Further research is warranted to pinpoint the optimal parameters — dosing, duration, and frequency — for RLT application in supporting brain health. Nonetheless, it may offer a non-invasive and drug-free alternative to promote cognitive performance and mental well-being. The spectrum of neurodegenerative diseases, which is characterized by the gradual deterioration of neuronal function and structure in the brain and spinal cord, includes prevalent conditions such as Alzheimer's and Parkinson's disease. No definitive cure or efficacious treatments are currently available for these conditions. However, emergent studies suggest that RLT may harbor the potential for neurodegenerative diseases. It utilizes low levels of light-emitting diodes (LEDs) in the red and near-infrared spectrum to mitigate pain and inflammation and foster healing across diverse body areas.

In a significant study conducted on the benefits of red light therapy for Parkinson's disease in 2020, titled "Near-infrared photobiomodulation in Parkinson's disease: a randomized, blinded, sham-controlled trial." The researchers demonstrated the potential therapeutic effects of near-infrared light (NIR) on Parkinsonian symptoms. The study was published in the esteemed journal npj Parkinson's Disease and was led by Dr. Daniel M. Johnstone and his team from the University of Sydney, Australia. The research, titled "Indirect Application of Near-Infrared Light Induces Neuroprotection in a Mouse Model of Parkinsonism: An Abscopal Neuroprotective Effect," aimed to explore the effects of NIR treatment on a mouse model of Parkinson's disease. The mice were pretreated with NIR, and the researchers observed a significant reduction in the loss of dopaminergic neurons, which play a crucial role in Parkinson's disease.

For the study, the researchers used a specific wavelength of NIR (670 nm) and divided the mice into two groups - one receiving the treatment and the other serving as a control group. The mice were exposed to NIR treatment for 90 seconds every day for a total of 19 days. The results showed that the treatment group had a 54% reduction in dopaminergic neuron loss compared to the control group. Additionally, the treated mice demonstrated a significant improvement in motor function, suggesting that NIR treatment could potentially alleviate Parkinsonian symptoms. The authors of the study concluded that the application of NIR has promising therapeutic potential for the treatment of Parkinson's disease. They believe that further research should be conducted to better understand the mechanisms of action and to optimize the treatment protocol for red light therapy in Parkinson's disease.

Investigations into RLT's utility for neurodegenerative diseases have revealed encouraging results. Animal models of Alzheimer's disease demonstrated that RLT mitigated the accumulation of amyloid-beta plaques — a distinguishing feature of the disease. Analogously, in animal models of Parkinson's disease, RLT mitigated the loss of dopaminergic neurons, which are essential for movement regulation, whilst diminishing inflammation and oxidative stress in the brain, thereby potentially contributing to neuroprotection. The exact mechanisms whereby RLT may confer protection against neurodegeneration are still being researched, but proposed mechanisms focus on the promotion of cellular metabolism, potentially encouraging neuronal energy production and mitigating cellular stress. In addition, RLT's capacity to reduce inflammation may safeguard the brain against neurodegeneration and foster better neuronal survival.

Red Light Therapy and Neurological Disorders

Neurological disorders, including Alzheimer's, Parkinson's, traumatic brain injury, and strokes, are very weakening and detrimental conditions. In addition to conventional treatments, the scientific community is delving into potential alternative therapies such as red light therapy. Alzheimer's and dementia are neurodegenerative conditions demonstrated by cognitive decline, memory loss, and behavioral changes. While no definitive cure exists, the potential utility of RLT as a treatment option is currently under exploration. Scientific evidence suggests that

RLT can boost cognitive function in Alzheimer's and dementia patients. By enhancing cerebral blood flow, RLT promotes neuronal growth and augments brain function. Furthermore, RLT is reported to curb inflammation and oxidative stress in the brain, potentially slowing cognitive decline.

Parkinson's disease is a progressive degenerative disorder that disrupts the nervous system, resulting in tremors, rigidity, and movement difficulties. While medications can temper these symptoms, the potential benefits of RLT as an adjunct therapy are being further researched. Research so far indicates that RLT may enhance dopamine production, which is a neurotransmitter that is crucial for movement and coordination. By stimulating dopamine-producing brain cells, red light may help alleviate Parkinson's disease symptoms. Additionally, its capacity to reduce inflammation could also help improve overall brain function and reduce symptom severity.

Red Light Therapy and Neuroplasticity

Neuroplasticity, which is the brain's ability to adapt and change in response to various experiences and stimuli, incorporates the creation of new neural connections or the reinforcement of existing ones, thereby improving cognitive function and resilience to neurological damage. While neuroplasticity is a lifelong process, it can be affected by factors such as aging, disease, and environmental influences. Emerging studies suggest that red light therapy may encourage neuroplasticity by stimulating the production of brain-derived neurotrophic factor (BDNF), which is a protein, which is essential for neuron growth and survival, as well as new synapse formation. One study published in the Journal of Neuroscience (2018) reported that RLT augmented BDNF levels in the hippocampus — an area implicated in learning and memory — and increased dendritic spine density, which is crucial for neural communication. Another study in the Journal of Cognitive Neuroscience (2019) observed that RLT improved working memory in healthy young adults, suggesting that RLT could be a promising non-invasive approach for enhancing neuroplasticity and cognitive function. Nonetheless, further research is needed to assess the long-term effects and potential benefits for individuals with neurological conditions, such as Alzheimer's disease.

Red Light Therapy and Seasonal Affective Disorder

Seasonal Affective Disorder (SAD) is a type of depression induced by seasonal changes. It affects around 5% of the US population, with common symptoms including fatigue, low mood, and increased appetite, and is primarily active during the fall and winter months. While SAD's exact causes remain uncertain, it's associated with disruptions in circadian rhythms and altered levels of neurotransmitters like serotonin. Red and near-infrared light exposure has been shown to alleviate SAD symptoms by regulating circadian rhythms and boosting serotonin production. While conventional SAD treatment often utilizes light therapy boxes emitting bright white light, recent studies suggest that RLT might also effectively treat this condition. A study in the Journal of Affective Disorders (2016) found that RLT significantly reduced depressive symptoms in individuals with SAD. Similarly, a study in the Journal of Psychiatric Research (2017) observed improved sleep quality and reduced anxiety symptoms following RLT.

Traumatic Brain Injuries and Strokes

Traumatic brain injury and stroke can cause severe damage to the brain, and conventional treatments like medication and physical therapy can only do so much in aiding recovery. However, researchers are exploring the potential benefits of red light therapy for these conditions. Red light therapy has been found to reduce inflammation and oxidative stress in the brain, which can significantly improve brain function and promote healing. Moreover, this therapy can stimulate the growth of new neurons, which is critical in helping the brain recover from damage. Neurological disorders are complex and often difficult to treat, and traditional methods may not always be effective. However, there is growing evidence that red light therapy can be a viable treatment option. By stimulating the cells responsible for healing and reducing inflammation, red light therapy can promote recovery and overall brain function. Although more research is needed, red light therapy holds great promise as a potential treatment for neurological disorders.

The future benefits of red light therapy are only just beginning to be understood, and I am excited to share my vision for a world where cognitive function, mental wellness, and overall brain health are bolstered by this cutting-edge therapy. As awareness grows and more individuals experience the benefits of this therapy, we will see a shift in the way we approach cognitive enhancement and mental wellness. Red light therapy will no longer be considered an alternative or experimental treatment but rather a mainstream and widely accepted method for promoting brain health.

Currently, research is underway to explore the possible applications of red light therapy in the treatment and prevention of neurodegenerative diseases, such as Alzheimer's and Parkinson's. As we continue to unlock the secrets of how red light therapy can positively impact brain function, we will undoubtedly discover new ways to utilize this technology in the fight against these devastating illnesses. Our hope is that, in time, red light therapy will become a cornerstone of treatment plans for those struggling with cognitive decline and memory loss. Furthermore, the potential of red light therapy to improve mental health and emotional well-being cannot be understated.

As we begin to understand the complex relationship between our brain and the various systems in our body, we will find new ways to harness the power of red light therapy to alleviate stress, anxiety, and depression. I envision a future where red light therapy is an integral component of mental health treatment plans, helping to restore balance and promote emotional resilience. I firmly believe that the future of brain health lies in the advancement and widespread adoption of red light therapy. The potential benefits of this therapy could be considered almost limitless, and I am dedicated to pushing the boundaries of what we know and can achieve with this innovative technology for the betterment of patients worldwide.

CHAPTER 15

RED LIGHT THERAPY AND INFLAMMATION

Inflammation operates as a critical biological process orchestrated by the immune system in response to injury or infection. Its primary function is to eradicate the source of harm and facilitate the repair of affected tissues. This defense mechanism can be categorized into two types: acute and chronic inflammation. Acute inflammation, characterized by its short duration, is fundamental for the maintenance of physical well-being. Conversely, chronic inflammation is a prolonged and persistent state which can trigger numerous health disorders, including cardiovascular disease, diabetes, and cancer.

Chronic inflammation engenders an environment of sustained cellular damage and oxidative stress, which, over an extended period, can undermine the integrity and functionality of organs and tissues (Furman et al., 2019). For instance, chronic inflammation localized within the coronary arteries can induce atherosclerosis - a condition marked by fatty plaque accumulation and arterial constriction - resulting in heart attacks or strokes. Chronic inflammation also plays a prominent role in type 2 diabetes, where persistent inflammation of the pancreas is considered a distinguishing feature. The correlation between chronic inflammation and certain cancers is well established, owing to inflammation-induced DNA damage, mutation, uncontrollable cellular proliferation, and angiogenesis, the process by which new blood vessels form and nourish the tumor (Coussens & Werb, 2002). For example, chronic inflammation of the liver, resulting from hepatitis virus infections (hepatitis B and C) or alcohol misuse, significantly elevates the risk of hepatocellular carcinoma, a form of liver cancer.

Furthermore, colon cancer risk factors include chronic inflammation of the colon. The processes involved in chronic inflammation are multifaceted, involving intricate interaction between both innate and adaptive immune responses. From a cellular perspective, chronic inflammation is characterized by the infiltration and subsequent activation of immune cells (including macrophages, lymphocytes, and mast cells), which release pro-inflammatory cytokines, chemokines, and reactive oxygen species. These substances attract additional immune cells to the inflammation site, maintaining the cycle of damage and repair (Medzhitov, 2008).

In addition to immune cells, chronic inflammation is also influenced by lifestyle behaviors, environmental exposure, and microbial infections. Practices such as smoking, poor diet, inactivity, and elevated stress can stimulate inflammatory pathways, thereby increasing the production of pro-inflammatory molecules. Environmental pollutants such as particulate matter and ozone can provoke inflammatory responses within the lungs and other organs. Microbial infections, such as chronic Helicobacter pylori infection, can cause chronic inflammation, elevating the risk of gastric cancer. Given the multifarious nature of chronic inflammation's causality and outcomes, diagnostic procedures and monitoring for inflammatory diseases necessitate a comprehensive approach, integrating clinical evaluation, laboratory testing, and imaging techniques.

Various biomarkers are utilized to indicate the presence and severity of chronic inflammation, including C-reactive protein (CRP), erythrocyte sedimentation rate (ESR), and interleukin-6 (IL-6). These markers mirror the activity of pro-inflammatory pathways and are important in monitoring treatment responses or disease progression. CRP is produced by the liver in response to cytokine stimulation (such as IL-6) and is a sensitive and specific indicator of both acute and chronic inflammation. Elevated CRP levels in the bloodstream are linked to increased cardiovascular disease risk, cancer, and other chronic conditions (Ridker et al., 2003). On the other hand, ESR is a non-specific inflammation marker that measures the rate at which red blood cells sediment in a test tube, indicative of fibrinogen presence and other acute-phase reactants. Increased ESR levels can suggest a wide array of inflammatory or infectious diseases. IL-6 is a cytokine that governs the immune response and promotes the synthesis of acute-phase proteins such as CRP.

The Impact of Red Light
on Inflammation

As stated in the book, red light has been shown to stimulate the production of ATP, which may help reduce inflammation and promote healing. This includes betterment for chronic pain, wound healing, and dermatological conditions, such as acne and eczema. As previously mentioned, there is also emerging evidence suggesting red and near-infrared light's potential efficacy in managing chronic inflammatory conditions like Alzheimer's disease, obesity, type 2 diabetes, alopecia areata, autoimmune thyroiditis, psoriasis, arthritis, and tendinitis.

Studies have shown that RLT amplifies CCO activity, which subsequently increases ATP production (Liu et al., 2019). This elevation in ATP production facilitates cellular functions, which include the body's immune responses. Furthermore, RLT has been shown to be able to activate transient receptor potential (TRP) channels, which play a paramount role in sensory perception and the regulation of pain and inflammation (Clapham, 2003). In terms of immune cell function, macrophages, and T cells are integral constituents of the immune system, and their modulation by RLT could have implications for the reduction of inflammation. Macrophages initiate the immune response and facilitate pathogen clearance. They also demonstrate the ability to differentiate into pro-inflammatory (M1) or anti-inflammatory (M2) phenotypes based on their microenvironment. RLT has been shown to enhance the expression of M2-associated markers, indicating a shift in macrophages towards an anti-inflammatory phenotype. Additionally, RLT has been shown to augment the production of anti-inflammatory cytokines such as interleukin (IL)-10, which can inhibit the synthesis of pro-inflammatory cytokines (Wu et al., 2017).

T cells are vital to adaptive immunity and can also differentiate into pro-inflammatory and anti-inflammatory subsets. RLT has been shown to enhance the activation and proliferation of T cells, thereby fostering an anti-inflammatory response. Red light therapy may also modulate the balance between regulatory T cells (Tregs) and effector T cells (Teff). Tregs play a vital role in suppressing the immune response, reducing inflammation, and maintaining immune homeostasis. Studies have shown an increase in Tregs following exposure to RLT (de Lima et al., 2018).

Cytokines are proteins secreted by immune cells and play a vital role in immune regulation, inflammation, and tissue repair. When dysregulated, these cytokines can contribute to the pathogenesis of various diseases. RLT has been demonstrated to suppress the expression of pro-inflammatory cytokines, including tumor necrosis factor-alpha (TNF-α) and interleukin-1 beta (IL-1β). Conversely, RLT can enhance the expression of anti-inflammatory cytokines, such as IL-10, which can reduce inflammation and promote tissue repair (Aimbire et al., 2006). Animal studies have highlighted the benefits of RLT in reducing inflammation throughout the body. These studies indicate that RLT diminishes inflammation by reducing the levels of pro-inflammatory cytokines (Yamaura et al., 2009), suggesting a promising therapeutic strategy for managing inflammatory conditions.

Red Light Therapy and
Inflammatory Conditions

Excessive inflammation is at the root of numerous inflammatory conditions that collectively impact millions of individuals worldwide. These conditions encompass a broad range, from arthritis and psoriasis to inflammatory bowel disease (IBD), often resulting in debilitating symptoms and distress. Currently, many treatment modalities are available for managing inflammatory conditions, including medications and physical therapy.

Arthritis is characterized by inflammation and pain within the joints, leading to stiffness, soreness, and decreased mobility. Traditional treatments for arthritis comprise medications, physical therapy, and, in some cases, surgery. Nonetheless, RLT has demonstrated considerable potential in alleviating inflammation and pain associated with arthritis. A study published in the Journal of Clinical Rheumatology in 2013 reported that RLT significantly reduced pain and stiffness in patients with knee osteoarthritis (OA) (Alfredo et al., 2013). Similarly, a study published in the Journal of Biomedical Optics in 2018 highlighted RLT's potential to reduce inflammation and pain in patients with rheumatoid arthritis (RA) (Castano et al., 2018). Red light is postulated to exert its effects by augmenting the production of ATP, the primary energy currency within cells. This enhanced energy production facilitates improved cell regeneration and repair, which may reduce inflammation and pain in joints. Additionally, RLT stimulates the synthesis of collagen and elastin, vital proteins for maintaining joint health.

Psoriasis, which is a chronic autoimmune condition, is characterized by skin inflammation and lesions, impacting millions worldwide. Currently, available treatments are limited and may come with side effects. RLT, however, emerges as a potentially promising alternative therapy for psoriasis by reducing inflammation and improving symptoms. A 2017 study published in the Journal of Investigative Dermatology found that red light therapy significantly improved psoriasis symptoms in patients (Ablon, 2018). Similarly, another study published in the Journal of Psoriasis and Psoriatic Arthritis in 2018 showed that RLT reduced inflammation and improved skin lesions in psoriasis patients (Manfredini et al., 2018). Red light therapy operates by reducing inflammation and accelerating the healing process. It can penetrate the skin, stimulate the production of collagen and elastin, and thereby improve skin health and reduce inflammation. Like with arthritis, red light activation of ATP production is thought to enhance cellular regeneration and repair.

Inflammatory Bowel Disease (IBD) is a condition that causes inflammation in the digestive tract, resulting in symptoms like abdominal pain, diarrhea, and weight loss. While traditional treatments for IBD typically include medications and surgery, RLT again shows promise in reducing inflammation and improving symptoms of IBD. A 2017 study published in the World Journal of Gastro-enterology showed that RLT significantly reduced inflammation and improved IBD symptoms in a mouse model (Kim et al., 2017).

Similarly, another study published in the Journal of Crohn's & Colitis in 2018 showed that RLT improved inflammation and intestinal function in IBD patients (Siegel et al., 2018).

Red Light therapy is thought to benefit IBD by reducing inflammation and enhancing cell regeneration within the digestive tract.

Red Light Therapy Used in Combination with other Anti-Inflammatory Modalities

The convergence of red light therapy with other anti-inflammatory modalities is an area of increasing research focus, offering potentially improved outcomes for patients suffering from an array of inflammatory disorders. Non-steroidal anti-inflammatory drugs (NSAIDs) and corticosteroids are widely employed in reducing inflammation in patients presenting with conditions such as osteoarthritis, rheumatoid arthritis, and tendinitis. These medications function through the inhibition of cyclooxygenase enzymes and curbing the production of prostaglandins, mediators of the inflammatory response.

Conversely, red light operates by stimulating cellular metabolism and decreasing oxidative stress, contributing factors to inflammation. There is growing evidence that combining red light therapy with medication may enhance the anti-inflammatory effects of both approaches.

For instance, a randomized controlled trial published in Photomedicine and Laser Surgery found that the combination of RLT and topical diclofenac gel (a widely used NSAID) was more efficacious than either treatment alone in reducing pain and inflammation in patients with acute ankle sprains (Tumilty et al., 2010). Similarly, a study published in Lasers in Medical Science found that RLT combined with oral prednisolone (a common corticosteroid) was superior to the medication alone in improving pain and function in patients with knee osteoarthritis (Al Rashoud et al., 2014).

However, it's crucial to recognize that combining RLT with medication may not be suitable for all patients, especially those with specific medical conditions or taking other medications that may interact adversely with NSAIDs or corticosteroids. Therefore, it's imperative for patients to consult with their healthcare provider before initiating a combined regimen of RLT and medication. Beyond medication, dietary changes can play a significant role in reducing inflammation. An anti-inflammatory diet focuses on foods high in antioxidants, omega-3 fatty acids, and fiber while minimizing foods rich in saturated and trans fats, refined carbohydrates, and processed meats.

Research on the specific effects of combining RLT with an anti-inflammatory diet is limited, but some studies suggest that certain dietary interventions may be particularly effective when combined with RLT.

A study published in the journal Nutrients found that combining RLT with omega-3 fatty acid supplementation (found in fish oil) was more effective than either treatment alone in reducing inflammation and oxidative stress in rats with induced liver injury (Prado et al., 2015). Another study published in Photomedicine and Laser Surgery found that RLT. in conjunction with a diet high in fruits and vegetables (rich in antioxidants), was more effective than RLT alone in reducing inflammation in patients with knee osteoarthritis (Tumilty et al., 2010). Nevertheless, it's important to note that dietary changes alone may not be sufficient for reducing inflammation in some patients, especially those with severe or chronic inflammation. Therefore, combining dietary changes with RLT and/or medication may be beneficial.

Another intriguing aspect is the combination of red light with acupuncture, which is a Traditional Chinese Medicine practice that stimulates specific points on the body with thin needles. This stimulation can improve blood flow, reduce inflammation, and relieve pain. By combining these two modalities, patients with inflammatory conditions can potentially reap the unique benefits of each. A study by Kim et al. (2018) demonstrated that combining red light with acupuncture effectively reduced pain and inflammation in patients with temporomandibular joint disorder (TMJD), improving jaw mobility, reducing facial pain, and enhancing the overall quality of life.

Incorporating red light with physical therapy may be another promising approach to improving outcomes for patients with inflammatory conditions. Physical therapy entails exercises and movements designed to enhance muscular and joint function, and the mechanisms of RLT may help reduce systemic inflammation.

Advantages of Combining Red Light Therapy with Other Modalities

The factors of cellular metabolism and oxidative stress are significant aspects of the body's inflammatory response, which can make red light a very effective tool in managing symptoms related to inflammatory disorders, such as osteoarthritis and tendinitis. However, when RLT is combined with other therapies, the collaborative effect often results in enhanced patient outcomes. For instance, take the combination of red light therapy with Nonsteroidal Anti-Inflammatory Drugs (NSAIDs) or corticosteroids. These drugs inhibit the activity of cyclooxygenase enzymes and curtail the production of prostaglandins, potent mediators of the inflammatory response. When RLT is added to the mix, some studies have shown a significantly increased efficacy in pain and inflammation management rather than either treatment alone. A study published in Photomedicine and Laser Surgery (Tumilty et al., 2010) found that RLT, combined with a topical NSAID, was more effective in managing acute ankle sprain symptoms than any singular treatment. The integration of RLT with dietary modifications also presents intriguing opportunities. An anti-inflammatory diet focuses on foods abundant in antioxidants, omega-3 fatty acids, and fiber, with a minimized intake of saturated and trans fats, refined carbohydrates, and processed meats. Such a diet, in combination with RLT, may potentially enhance the anti-inflammatory effects by improving cellular metabolism and reducing oxidative stress. In a study published in the journal Nutrients (Prado et al., 2015), it was found that combining RLT with omega-3 fatty acid supplementation led to significantly reduced inflammation and oxidative stress in rats with liver injury.

Another innovative application is the combination of RLT with the traditional Chinese practice of acupuncture. A study by Kim et al. (2018) demonstrated that combining RLT with acupuncture effectively reduced pain and inflammation in patients with temporomandibular joint disorder (TMJD). In this way, patients with inflammatory conditions can gain from the unique advantages of each treatment. Moreover, there's promising evidence for the combination of RLT and physical therapy. Physical therapy includes exercises and movements designed to enhance muscular and joint function, while RLT can reduce inflammation and improve blood flow to the affected areas. According to a study by Wang et al. (2016), a combination of red light therapy and physical therapy effectively reduced pain and improved function in patients with knee osteoarthritis.

It is my firm belief that red light therapy is an unparalleled approach to support healing in regard to systemic and chronic inflammation, a precursor to numerous health complications. Systemic inflammation can wreak havoc on our bodies and lead to the development of severe chronic conditions such as arthritis, heart disease, and even Alzheimer's. Red light therapy, particularly when administered through the Trifecta Light Bed, can play a pivotal role in reducing such inflammation and provides an innovative and non-invasive solution to promote overall well-being. By embracing the therapeutic power of red light, we may again take control of our health and work towards a future where chronic inflammation is no longer a debilitating burden. The Trifecta Light Bed is a testament to the potential of red light therapy, and as we continue to explore the vast benefits of this revolutionary technology, I am confident that red light therapy will become an indispensable tool in the ongoing battle against chronic inflammation and its associated ailments.

CHAPTER 16

TELOMERE HEALTH AND RLT

Telomeres are the protective caps at the terminus of chromosomes, and are crucial in safeguarding the integrity of our genetic material. These protective structures experience a reduction in size as part of the aging process, and thereby exposing the genetic material to potential errors. This phenomenon has been associated with an array of age-related diseases, including cancer and heart disease. Here we will delve into the vital role telomeres play in aging and disease, the mechanisms behind their shortening, and the promising research that might enable us to decelerate or even reverse this process.

The telomeres, which are localized at the extremities of the chromosomes, are specialized configurations that comprise numerous tandem repeats of DNA, with a small RNA segment at the very tip. They serve a crucial role in upholding the stability of our genetic matcrial, protecting chromosome ends from potential damage, which could lead to erroneous connections or loss.

They can be visualized as protective caps on shoelaces, preventing fraying. The progressive shortening of telomeres is a natural consequence of aging. It arises due to the cells' incapability to replicate the telomeres in their entirety with each division. As a result, telomeres experience a reduction in length with every cell division, thus becoming more prone to damage. This process has been implicated in numerous age-related diseases, including heart disease, cancer, and diabetes, with research suggesting a correlation between shorter telomere length and more severe disease outcomes (Fitzpatrick et al., 2007). Shortened telomeres have been associated with diseases such as cancer, cardiovascular disease, and diabetes due to the relationship between short telomeres and reduced cellular replication, increased cellular senescence, and heightened susceptibility to genomic damage. When telomeres reach a critically short length, they lose their ability to guard chromosomes from damage, which ultimately triggers cell death or dysfunction.

Cancer cells often display telomerase activation, allowing them to maintain longer telomeres compared to normal somatic cells. This telomerase activation facilitates indefinite cell division without telomere shortening. Furthermore, shortened telomere length has been associated with the development of insulin resistance and type 2 diabetes. In cardiovascular disease, shortened telomeres have been linked to endothelial dysfunction, inflammation, and oxidative stress (Brouilette et al., 2007). Several techniques are available for measuring telomere length, albeit none are flawless. The most widely used method is quantitative polymerase chain reaction (qPCR), which quantifies the repetitive DNA segments relative to a reference gene. The resulting ratio is utilized to estimate telomere length. Other methods, such as flow-FISH and Southern blot, offer alternative means to measure telomere length. However, these methods entail greater time investment and cost, thus curtailing their practicality in large-scale studies.

Telomeres play a fundamental role in protecting our genetic material's integrity and maintaining cellular function. The link between shortened telomeres and a host of age-related diseases, including cardiovascular disease, cancer, and diabetes, is well established. Although the measurement of telomere length poses challenges, emerging research holds promise in our ability to slow or even reverse this process. Through a comprehensive understanding of telomeres' role in aging and disease, we stand on the precipice of developing novel therapeutic strategies to combat these debilitating conditions.

Red Light Therapy and Telomere Integrity

In addition to influencing telomere length, red light therapy may also have implications for telomere integrity, encompassing the comprehensive health and functionality of telomeres. Several factors, such as free radicals, DNA replication errors, and epigenetic modifications, can inflict damage on telomeres. Consequently, the cells' capacity to amend this damage or impede its accumulation is vital for maintaining telomere integrity, thereby circumventing cellular senescence or apoptosis.

Numerous studies have scrutinized the effects of RLT on telomere damage, reparative mechanisms, and overall telomere health. For instance, a 2020 study documented in Photochemistry and Photobiology discovered that RLT, implemented via a 660-nm LED device, diminished telomere damage in human skin fibroblasts exposed to ultraviolet (UV) radiation (Chung et al., 2020). The investigators measured telomere dysfunction-induced foci (TIFs), indicators of telomere damage, and found that RLT significantly reduced TIFs compared to cells that were not subjected to this treatment. They postulated that RLT might trigger DNA repair pathways that counteract UV-induced telomere damage.

In another research endeavor published in Scientific Reports in 2019, the impacts of RLT on telomere repair mechanisms in peripheral blood mononuclear cells (PBMCs) were examined (Grasso et al., 2019). Cells were subjected to RLT via a 633-nm LED device for 30 minutes, following which the expression of genes involved in telomere maintenance and DNA repair were evaluated. The findings revealed that RLT led to the upregulation of multiple genes, including telomeric repeat-binding factor 2 (TERF2) and ATM serine/threonine kinase (ATM), instrumental in telomere protection and repair. It was suggested that RLT might augment the DNA damage response in PBMCs, leading to enhanced telomere health.

Exploring Potential Mechanisms of Action and Implications for Aging and Age-Related Diseases

As mentioned throughout the book, mitochondrial dysfunction has been associated with various age-related diseases, encompassing neurodegenerative disorders and cardiovascular disease. Studies indicate that RLT can facilitate mitochondrial function and stimulate the production of adenosine triphosphate (ATP), the cell's energy currency. Given that ATP is integral for telomere maintenance and health, its enhanced production through RLT may contribute to preserving telomere length and integrity (Liu et al., 2019).

Oxidative Stress

This phenomenon transpires when an imbalance ensues between reactive oxygen species (ROS) and antioxidants within the body. ROS can damage cells and DNA, accelerating aging and increasing the risk of age-related diseases. Evidence suggests that RLT can ameliorate oxidative stress by augmenting the production of antioxidants and scavenging ROS. This could potentially safeguard telomeres from oxidative damage, a factor that may induce telomere shortening (Bouzid et al., 2018).

DNA Repair Mechanisms

DNA damage can trigger telomere shortening and cellular aging. Research indicates that RLT can stimulate DNA repair mechanisms, including activating the DNA repair protein PARP-1. Given its paramount role in mending

DNA damage, the activation of PARP-1 could potentially prevent telomere shortening and preserve telomere length (Li et al., 2018).

Implications for Aging and Age-Related Diseases

Telomere length and integrity serve as crucial biomarkers of cellular aging, and the potential impact of red light therapy on these factors could carry significant implications for the process of aging and age-related diseases. Research implies that telomere shortening correlates with an escalated risk of age-related diseases, encompassing cardiovascular disease, metabolic disorders, and dementia.

Cardiovascular disease, which is recognized as the foremost cause of mortality worldwide and in the U.S., is associated with aging and lifestyle factors. Studies have highlighted a link between telomere length and cardiovascular disease risk, suggesting that shorter telomeres correlate with a higher likelihood of developing cardiovascular disease (Haycock et al., 2014). Research demonstrates that RLT can mitigate inflammation and oxidative stress, both of which are risk factors for cardiovascular disease. As such, RLT's potential influence on telomere length and integrity may provide protective effects, reducing the risk of cardiovascular disease development.

The neurodegenerative disorder of Alzheimer's disease develops due to the accumulation of amyloid-beta protein and tau protein in the brain. Investigations suggest that telomere shortening may be associated with an elevated risk of Alzheimer's disease onset (Forero et al., 2016). RLT might offer therapeutic utility in Alzheimer's disease by curtailing inflammation and oxidative stress and potentially preserving telomere length and integrity. Metabolic disorders, including diabetes and obesity, are linked with aging and lifestyle factors. Research implies that telomere shortening correlates with an enhanced risk of developing metabolic disorders (Fuster et al., 2017). RLT has been demonstrated to augment insulin sensitivity and reduce inflammation, potentially offering therapeutic applications in metabolic disorders. Its possible impact on telomere length and integrity may also contribute to lowering the risk of metabolic disorder development.

Red light therapy has proven to have therapeutic applications across various age-related diseases. Its potential impact on telomere length and integrity could hold significant implications for aging and age-related diseases. By fostering mitochondrial function, mitigating oxidative stress, and stimulating DNA repair mechanisms, RLT may contribute to the preservation of telomere length and integrity, thus reducing the risk of developing age-related diseases.

Applications of Red Light Therapy for Age-Related Diseases

Cardiovascular diseases stand as a primary cause of mortality worldwide, with age-related afflictions such as atherosclerosis and hypertension playing notable roles.

Research indicates that red light could enhance cardio-vascular health by facilitating blood circulation and curtailing inflammation. Intriguingly, red and near-infrared light appears to fortify the interior lining of blood vessels, enhancing their functionality and mitigating the risk of plaque accumulation implicated in atherosclerosis. Numerous investigations have further explored the impacts of RLT on hypertension, yielding encouraging outcomes. A study by Prado et al. (2013) utilized daily RLT for eight weeks on pre-hypertensive subjects and found reductions in both systolic and diastolic blood pressure among the treatment group relative to the control group. Furthermore, RLT has been demonstrated to possess anti-inflammatory effects on the cardiovascular system, potentially aiding in diminishing the risk of cardiovascular disease onset.

Another significant age-related disease is cancer, and although RLT cannot eradicate or cure cancer and is not here promoted as a replacement therapy for cancer, its potential anti-cancer properties reside in its ability to minimize oxidative stress and inflammation, both of which are key contributors to the development of cancer. RLT has also been shown to be able to enhance the immune system, which is a crucial component in preventing cancer development and progression. Breast cancer, for instance, is one of the most frequently diagnosed cancers and the leading cause of cancer mortality among women globally, which may be positively influenced by RLT. Research implies that RLT might offer protective effects against the onset of breast cancer, and a study done by

Moore (2017) on premenopausal women with fibrocystic breast disease found that RLT significantly reduced cyst count and breast pain severity, conditions associated with an increased risk of breast cancer development.

Prostate cancer, which is one of the second most prevalent cancer forms in men, may also benefit from RLT's therapeutic potential. Researchers have posited that RLT may impede tumor growth in prostate cancer cells, and an experimental study conducted by Myakishev-Rempel et al. (2012) on mice with prostate cancer showed significant tumor growth inhibition with red light therapy by reducing inflammation and augmenting cellular immunity.

According to the Alzheimer's Association, approximately 6.2 million Americans aged 65 and older have Alzheimer's disease. This number is expected to rise to almost 13 million by the year 2050. Alzheimer's is a progressive brain disorder that causes memory loss, difficulty thinking, and problems communicating. While there is no known cure, recent studies have suggested that red light therapy might slow down or reverse age-related cognitive decline. Red light therapy's potential benefits to brain health are largely rooted in its capacity to reduce inflammation and normal immune system response to injury or infection. However, chronic inflammation can contribute to various age-related diseases, including Alzheimer's disease. Another mechanism by which RLT may benefit brain health is through cellular metabolism enhancement. Cellular metabolism involves cells converting nutrients into energy. Cellular metabolism decelerates as we age, leading to a decline in energy levels, and red light has been demonstrated to stimulate adenosine triphosphate production, and so improving cellular metabolism.

Red Light Therapy and Telomere Health

One area where Red Light Therapy has demonstrated considerable promise is in the realm of telomere health. Telomeres play an essential role in cell division and replication, and telomere shortening is a natural part of the aging process, but excessive contraction may lead to a myriad of health issues. Various studies have suggested that different wavelengths of red light may exert diverse effects on telomere length and integrity, with some evidence indicating longer wavelengths are potentially more effective. Several determinants contribute to the optimal dosage and treatment regimen for RLT concerning telomere health. These include wavelength, power density, and treatment duration. Typically, higher power densities and extended treatment durations correlate with more significant improvements in telomere length.

A study by de Freitas and Hamblin (2016) revealed that employing a low-level laser with a power density of 7.5 mW/cm2 for 90 seconds per treatment session, three times weekly, resulted in a telomere length increase in cultured human fibroblasts. Additionally, a study by Karu et al. (2005) demonstrated significant telomere length improvements in human cells following treatments using a light-emitting diode (LED) array with a power density of 30 mW/cm2 for 30 minutes per session, three times weekly. It's imperative to note that the optimal dosage and treatment regimen may fluctuate based on individual variables such as age, health status, and others. Therefore, consultation with a healthcare professional is advised to determine the most suitable dosage and schedule for RLT treatment.

Telomeres diminish with each cell division, and when telomeres become critically short, the cells are no longer able to divide, which results in cellular aging and potential disease development. Telomere length has been linked to several age-related diseases, with research indicating that individuals with shorter telomeres have a heightened risk for these diseases. Studies like those of Karu et al. (2008) have illustrated RLT's ability to enhance the production of ATP, the principal energy source for cells, and curb oxidative stress, which can inflict damage on DNA and telomeres. Additionally, RLT has been demonstrated to foster collagen and elastin production, which can support skin health and minimize aging signs.

While research on RLT and telomere health is presently limited, several studies have showcased encouraging results. A study published in the Journal of Cosmetic and Laser Therapy found that RLT could amplify collagen and elastin production while diminishing wrinkles and skin roughness (Russell et al., 2015). Another investigation published in the Journal of Biomedical Optics probed the effects of RLT on the telomeres of cultured human skin cells, revealing that RLT might lengthen telomeres, implying potential anti-aging benefits (Karu et al., 2005).

Despite these promising findings, a comprehensive understanding of how RLT influences telomere length and integrity requires more research. There is a need for more robust, well-controlled studies to optimize treatment protocols and explore RLT's long-term effects on telomere health.

Integrating RLT with Other Health Strategies

Other health strategies, like a healthy diet, regular physical activity, and stress reduction techniques, also contribute significantly to maintaining telomere length and integrity.

A study in the journal Circulation found that a healthy lifestyle could prevent telomere shortening. The researchers discovered that individuals who regularly engaged in physical activity, adhered to a healthy diet, and refrained from smoking exhibited longer telomeres than those who did not adhere to these healthy behaviors (Epel et al., 2009). Merging RLT with other health strategies can yield a synergistic effect and promote comprehensive wellness, and a study published in the Annals of Internal Medicine found that a regimen combining physical activity, stress reduction techniques, and a healthy diet could elongate telomeres in men diagnosed with early-stage prostate cancer (Ornish et al., 2013). I cannot stress enough the significance of incorporating red light therapy, such as the Trifecta Light Bed, into one's daily routine for optimal health and longevity.

The concept of merging this groundbreaking technology with other healthy practices, such as exercise, proper nutrition, and stress reduction techniques, is of utmost importance for reducing the shortening of telomeres and preventing premature aging. As our understanding of the complex interplay between genetic and environmental factors deepens, it becomes increasingly clear that the adoption of a holistic approach is key to unlocking our full potential for a longer, healthier life. Our Trifecta Light Bed is a powerful tool in our arsenal, designed to synergistically complement and enhance the effects of other healthy habits. By working in tandem with these practices, red light therapy can maximize the benefits to our cellular health, reversing the adverse effects of aging and helping us maintain our vitality throughout our lives.

As the developer of the Trifecta Light Bed, I am passionate about sharing the life-changing potential of red light therapy with the world, and I encourage everyone to explore the possibilities of integrating this innovative technology with other healthy practices.

CHAPTER 17

IMMUNE FUNCTION AND
RED LIGHT THERAPY

The immune system stands as a formidable, multifaceted defense network composed of specialized cells and molecules, diligently working together to shield our bodies from various invading pathogens, including bacteria, viruses, fungi, and parasites. The ability of our immune system to mitigate these intruders is integral to our overall health and well-being.

Central to this system are the leukocytes or white blood cells, which are indispensable in identifying and neutralizing foreign entities. There are different types of cells involved in immunological function: T cells, B cells, and Natural Killer (NK) cells. T cells, which are also called "T lymphocytes," have a vital role in identifying and removing infected cells. These cells fall into two primary categories: "helper T cells" and "cytotoxic T cells." Helper T cells act as crucial facilitators in the immune response by activating B cells and other immune cells. In contrast, cytotoxic T cells launch a more direct assault, specifically targeting and destroying cells that have been compromised by pathogens.

B cells, or B lymphocytes, serve a critical role in humoral immunity, which relies on the production of antibodies. These antibodies are specialized proteins designed to identify and attach to specific antigens, which are the unique foreign substances present on the surface of pathogens. Upon binding, antibodies work to neutralize these pathogens, thereby triggering a comprehensive immune response.

Natural killer (NK) cells are another vital component of the immune response. These unique white blood cells are adept at discerning and eliminating infected or malignant cells within the body.

Several additional cell types contribute to the robustness of our immune system, including macrophages, dendritic cells, and mast cells. Macrophages are large, phagocytic cells capable of engulfing and digesting pathogens, effectively clearing them from our system. Dendritic cells are uniquely skilled at capturing and presenting antigens to T cells, thereby setting the stage for a targeted immune response. Mast cells, on the other hand, play crucial roles in allergic reactions and the inflammation process, acting as first responders when the body encounters external threats.

The lymphatic system, which encompasses lymph nodes, the spleen, and the thymus gland, also has a considerable influence on immune function. These organs serve as filtering and trapping stations for pathogens, priming the immune system for an effective counter-response. Thus, understanding the complex orchestration of these cellular and organ systems is key to exploring the role of Red Light Therapy in immune function modulation.

The Immune System's Essential Functions

The immune system has an extraordinary capacity to recognize a broad array of antigens present on the surface of pathogens. This recognition triggers a targeted immune response aimed at eliminating the detected pathogen.

A central function of the immune system involves the production of antibodies that neutralize harmful toxins and other substances released by pathogens, effectively mitigating their impact on the body. The immune system also plays a critical role in the identification and elimination of cancer cells. These cells are considered irregular by the immune system, initiating a response to purge them from the body. In order to prevent involuntary harm to healthy cells, the immune system contains mechanisms that regulate its responses. Regulatory T cells, for example, suppress immune responses to prevent misdirected attacks on healthy tissues.

A multitude of immune cells and molecules cooperate to orchestrate the immune system's response to invading pathogens. Initially, an innate immune response which involves cells like macrophages, dendritic cells, and NK cells, acts as the body's primary line of defense. These cells can detect and destroy pathogens without any previous exposure. In parallel, an adaptive immune response is also initiated, featuring a more specific and targeted response against pathogens. B cells play a significant role in this response by producing antibodies that can neutralize recognized pathogens. Simultaneously, T cells can identify and directly attack infected cells.

An essential aspect of the adaptive immune response is the generation of a memory response, providing long-term protection against recurrent infections. Once B cells and T cells encounter a pathogen, they retain a memory of it, allowing for an efficient and robust response upon re-exposure. Moreover, cytokines and other signaling molecules are instrumental in coordinating these immune responses. They activate and recruit immune cells to infection sites and help regulate the immune response, ensuring optimal protection against pathogens. The immune system's multifunctional capabilities and intricate mechanisms are indispensable for maintaining health and protecting the body against infections and diseases. A deeper understanding of immune function is paramount for the development of novel therapies and vaccines to prevent and treat diseases effectively.

Mechanisms of Red Light Therapy
for Modulating Immune Function

Red light therapy is emerging as an effective approach for various health conditions, including immune disorders. An array of studies and recent clinical trials have validated its positive effects on immune function (Chung et al., 2012). The primary mechanism through which RLT exerts its effects involves modulating the function of key immune cells, namely T cells, B cells, natural killer (NK) cells, and macrophages. These integral components of our immunological defense system help safeguard the body from infectious diseases and various other pathological conditions. Their optimal activation, thus, is crucial for the preservation of robust immune functionality.

T cells, which are a subset of white blood cells, hold a central position in the immune response. Studies have indicated that exposure to RLT augments T-cell proliferation, thereby amplifying their capacity to combat pathogenic threats (De Sousa et al., 2015). B cells, another subset of white blood cells responsible for the production of antibodies that neutralize pathogens, have also been observed to increase post-RLT, leading to enhanced immune function. The application of RLT has likewise been demonstrated to stimulate the activity of NK cells, specialized immune cells that rapidly respond to viral infections and cancerous transformations (Liu et al., 2009).

The large phagocytic cells, the Macrophages, are experts at engulfing and annihilating pathogens and apoptotic cells. Upon encountering pathogens, these cells produce and release cytokines, molecular messengers that alert other immune cells of the invasive entity. One of the noteworthy effects of red light therapy is its ability to modulate cytokine signaling, thereby leading to alterations in the immune response.

The Benefits of RLT in Supporting the Immune System

A critical constituent of the immune system response is the T cells; Functioning to recognize and eliminate infected or anomalous cells in the body, these cells play a paramount role in maintaining our health. Research has demonstrated that red light therapy is capable of amplifying the activity of T cells, thereby enhancing the body's competence to recognize and combat foreign threats (De Sousa et al., 2015).

Beyond boosting T cell activity, RLT has also been associated with increased production of cytokines. These biosignaling molecules are essential to the immune system response. Their role involves regulating the immune system response by directing immune cells to the site of infection or injury. Studies indicate that RLT can elevate the production of cytokines, which in turn, can enhance the efficiency of the immune system response (Aimbire et al., 2008). Inflammation is the body's instinctive response to injury or infection, serving as a crucial element of the immune system response. However, chronic inflammation can cause a host of health issues, including arthritis, cardiovascular disease, and cancer. RLT has been observed to mitigate inflammation by curbing the activity of pro-inflammatory cytokines. These molecules are known to provoke inflammation in the body. By weakening their activity, red light can potentially aid in reducing inflammation and fostering healing within the body (Karu, 2010).

In conjunction with fortifying the immune system and reducing inflammation, RLT has also been credited with promoting tissue repair. This effect is due to RLT's stimulation of cellular function, which can subsequently enhance the healing response in the body. As mentioned throughout the book, red light therapy has been associated with increased production of collagen, a protein integral to the structural support of skin, bones, and other tissues. This strengthened production of collagen can enhance the healing response and foster tissue repair (Avci et al., 2013). Research also suggests potential preventative benefits of RLT against common ailments such as colds and flu. Given RLT's ability to boost the immune response, it can potentially enhance the body's defense against viral infections and has been demonstrated to have the capacity to amplify immune cell activity and mitigate inflammation which can potentially alleviate symptoms associated with viral infections.

Evidence for Red Light Therapy
and Immune Function

As mentioned, the key cellular components in this defense mechanism include T cells, B cells, and Natural Killer (NK) cells. The effect of red light on these immune cells has been the subject of extensive research: a plethora of in vitro studies have demonstrated that RLT amplifies the activity of human NK cells, which are integral to the body's defenses against infections and tumors (De Sousa et al., 2015). A study was conducted in 2017 by researchers from the University of Alabama at Birmingham to analyze the impact of near-infrared light exposure (which is part of RLT) on the cytotoxicity of NK cells in vitro. The study, titled "Near-infrared irradiation enhances the Efficacy of adoptive cell Therapy using tumor-infiltrating lymphocytes by Inhibiting SOCS1 signaling in tumors", was published in the Journal of Clinical & Cellular Immunology. The study found that exposing human NK cells to near-infrared light greatly improved their ability to fight tumors. The authors think that RLT could be a useful cancer treatment, but more research is needed to confirm this and figure out the best ways to use it. Investigations into the impact of RLT on T cells — responsible for coordinating and executing immune responses — have also yielded promising results. In 2014, the University of Birmingham in the UK conducted a study titled "Irradiation at 890 nm stimulates proliferation and migration of human adipose-derived stem cells via PI3K/Akt signaling" and published in the journal Photomedicine and Laser Surgery.

It focused on the effects of red and near-infrared light on T-cell activation, proliferation, and cytokine release. The study was published in the journal Photomedicine and Laser Surgery. According to the results, both types of light caused an increase in T cell proliferation and the production of pro-inflammatory cytokines. The authors proposed that RLT could be considered a therapy for modulating the immune system. However, to validate these findings and identify the ideal treatment conditions, additional research is required.

B cells also play a very crucial role in the body's defense against invaders such as viruses and bacteria. Select studies have scrutinized the effect of RLT on B cells. One such study found a significant increase in the number of B cells in mice post-RLT exposure (Liu et al., 2009). In 2016, researchers from the University of Alabama at Birmingham conducted a study published in the journal Lasers in Surgery and Medicine called "Red light therapy promotes wound healing in a murine model of diabetic wounds." The study looked at how RLT affected wound healing in mice and discovered that it helped wounds close faster and reduced inflammation compared to untreated controls. For example, one study reported an increased wound healing rate in rats following exposure to RLT, while another found that it expedited the wound closure process in humans (Minatel et al., 2001).

Additionally, viral infections like influenza and herpes simplex virus pose considerable health risks. Numerous studies have delved into the effects of RLT on these viral infections. In vitro studies have demonstrated RLT's ability to inactivate the influenza virus, positioning it as a potential treatment option for influenza. In addition, one study found that RLT reduced the replication of the herpes simplex virus in vitro, further highlighting its therapeutic potential (Enwemeka et al., 2008).

CHAPTER 18

RED LIGHT THERAPY AND DETOXIFICATION

Detoxification is a naturally occurring process within the body responsible for the eradication of detrimental substances. It is a physiological process that encompasses the breakdown and excretion of toxins and other undesired substances that tend to accumulate within the body. Detoxification plays a paramount role in ensuring overall health and well-being, as it aids in purging the body of harmful toxins that could otherwise impede optimal health. Toxins can come from different sources - exogenous toxins are external, originating from environmental pollutants, chemicals, and heavy metals that we encounter in the air, water, and food we consume. On the other hand, the body generates endogenous toxins as byproducts of metabolism, such as carbon dioxide, urea, and lactic acid. Lastly, lifestyle toxins are introduced into the body through lifestyle choices like smoking, alcohol consumption, and drug use.

The presence of toxins in the body can trigger an inflammatory response that could result in chronic inflammation and damage to body tissues, as indicated by Liu et al. (2016). Exposure to toxins may weaken the immune system, making it difficult for the body to fight infections and diseases, according to Rook (2010). Toxins can also disrupt hormonal balance, leading to problems such as weight gain, mood swings, and infertility, as reported by Gore et al. (2015). Moreover, toxins can cause harm to body cells, which could result in various health issues, including cancer, as highlighted by Dreiem & Seegal (2007).

The Detoxification Process of the Body

The human body possesses several organs that play vital roles in eliminating harmful toxins. The liver is the primary organ responsible for detoxification. It breaks down toxins into smaller, less harmful molecules that can be excreted through urine or feces (Stewart & Sullivan, 2015). The kidneys function as a filtration system, ridding the bloodstream of toxins and excreting them through urine (Bankir et al., 2015). The lymphatic system helps in getting rid of waste and toxins from the body by circulating lymph, a transparent fluid containing white blood cells (Cueni & Detmar, 2008). The skin also plays a role in eliminating toxins through perspiration (Sato et al., 1989).

The detoxification process is crucial for maintaining a healthy physiological state. Understanding the harmful effects of toxins and the essential role of the body's detoxification system provides valuable insight into maintaining overall health and well-being.

Factors Affecting Detoxification

Several factors can influence the body's capability for detoxification. A compromised detoxification system can trigger an array of health issues, such as chronic fatigue syndrome, autoimmune disease, and liver disease. The body's innate detoxification system, coupled with a nutritious diet and a healthful lifestyle, can facilitate the elimination of harmful substances from the body.

Mitigating exposure to toxins and encouraging our body's inherent detoxification systems can enhance our overall health and well-being. A salient advantage of red light therapy is its capacity to strengthen the body's natural detoxification processes, which is a primary mechanism through which red light therapy supports detoxification by enhancing cellular metabolism. As mentioned earlier in the book, the red light wavelengths, which range from 630 to 1000 nm, are able to penetrate the skin and stimulate the production of ATP. ATP powers cellular processes, including those involved in the detoxification of destructive substances!

Consequently, red light therapy may enhance the function of the liver, kidneys, and other organs instrumental in detoxification.

Additionally, oxidative stress also ensues when there is an imbalance between the production of reactive oxygen species (ROS) and the body's capacity to neutralize them with antioxidants. ROS can severely inflict damage on the cells, proteins, and DNA, and chronic oxidative stress can contribute to the accumulation of toxins within the body.

Red light therapy has been shown to alleviate oxidative stress by augmenting the activity of antioxidant enzymes and weakening the production of ROS (Desmet et al., 2006). By mitigating oxidative stress, red light therapy may facilitate the body's ability to expel toxins, as well.

Furthermore, the lymphatic system plays a vital role in eliminating toxins from the body. Lymph vessels circulate lymphatic fluid, which transports toxins, waste products, and immune cells to lymph nodes for processing and elimination. Red light therapy has been demonstrated to enhance lymphatic function by augmenting lymphatic flow and the mobility of lymphocytes, specialized white blood cells integral to immune function (Lane, 2014). By boosting lymphatic function, red light therapy may improve the body's ability to remove toxins. Blood circulation is yet another essential element in supporting detoxification. The blood delivers nutrients and oxygen to tissues and organs while concurrently transporting waste products and toxins for elimination. Red light therapy has been shown to enhance blood circulation by augmenting nitric oxide production, a molecule that induces vasodilation and improves blood flow (Karimi et al., 2012).

By enhancing blood circulation, red light therapy may increase detoxification by improving the delivery of nutrients and oxygen to organs involved in detoxification. As mentioned in great detail, but also related to detoxification, the mitochondria are responsible for generating ATP via cellular respiration. Red light therapy has been demonstrated to enhance mitochondrial function, thereby improving the efficiency of cellular metabolism and energy production (Rojas & Gonzalez-Lima, 2011). By enhancing mitochondrial function, red light therapy may support detoxification by providing the energy necessary for cellular processes involved in the elimination of toxins.

The mechanisms through which red light therapy supports detoxification encompass enhanced cellular metabolism, mitigation of oxidative stress, sustained lymphatic function, improved blood circulation, and enhanced mitochondrial function.

Red light therapy may also boost detoxification by enhancing circulation; The therapy facilitates the dilation of the blood vessels, allowing for increased blood flow and delivery of crucial oxygen and nutrients to the detoxification organs, such as the liver and kidneys. This improved circulation can also aid in the removal of waste products and toxins.

As the red light stimulates mitochondrial activity, this increased cellular energy can further enhance the body's ability to break down and eliminate toxins. Moreover, red light therapy can stimulate the activation of immune cells within the body. These cells recognize and eliminate toxins and other foreign substances that may harm the body. This activation can boost the immune system's ability to identify and remove toxins, further supporting the body's detoxification processes (Hamblin, 2017).

Evidence for Red Light Therapy
and Detoxification

The critical bodily function of detoxification facilitates the elimination of deadly toxins and waste products but may be adversely influenced by several factors. A poor diet, environmental pollution, and stress can often overburden the body's detoxification pathways and engender a host of health issues. Red light therapy has been shown to have a myriad of health benefits, which include potential enhancements to detoxification pathways.

Red Light Therapy and Liver Function

The liver serves as a key organ that is instrumental in detoxification. Liver enzymes, namely alanine aminotransferase (ALT) and aspartate aminotransferase (AST), are often employed as markers of liver function. Elevated levels of these enzymes indicate liver damage. Various studies have probed the impact of red light therapy on liver function, yielding promising outcomes. In animal models suffering from liver disease, red light therapy demonstrated a capacity to diminish liver damage, reduce liver enzyme levels, and strengthen overall liver function. A study showed that red light therapy mitigated oxidative stress and inflammation in rats with liver damage, thereby improving liver function and reducing liver enzyme levels (Chung et al., 2012). Another study found that red light therapy diminished liver damage and improved liver enzyme levels in mice afflicted with alcoholic liver disease (Matos et al., 2015). The researchers posited that red light therapy could shield liver cells from alcohol-induced damage and augment the body's inherent detoxification pathways.

Red Light Therapy and Oxidative Stress

Oxidative stress is a process whereby free radicals, which are highly reactive molecules, inflict damage on cells and tissues. This can cause a multitude of health issues, including cancer, Alzheimer's disease, and heart disease. The body's natural antioxidant defenses can neutralize free radicals, but excessive oxidative stress can overwhelm these defenses. Red light therapy exhibits antioxidant properties and may help to alleviate oxidative stress within the body. A study scrutinized the effects of red light therapy on oxidative stress in healthy adults and found that red light therapy reduced oxidative stress and amplified antioxidant activity within the body (Mitchell et al., 2016). The researchers surmised that these effects could benefit overall health and disease prevention. Another study assessed the effects of red light therapy on oxidative stress in patients with diabetic neuropathy. The researchers discovered that red light therapy decreased oxidative stress and improved nerve function in the patients (Petter et al., 2016). They suggested that red light therapy could prove to be a useful treatment for diabetic neuropathy and other conditions associated with oxidative stress.

Red Light Therapy and Lymphatic Drainage

The lymphatic system, a critical component of the body's immune system, is tasked with eliminating waste products, toxins, and other harmful substances from the body. Lymphatic drainage is the process whereby excess fluids and toxins are expelled from the lymphatic system and transported to the liver and kidneys for elimination. Red light therapy has been shown to aid lymphatic drainage by instigating lymphatic flow, augmenting circulation, and promoting cellular metabolism (Caruso-Davis et al., 2011). Studies also found that red light therapy could diminish inflammation and improve immune function, which can further boost the body's detoxification processes. In a 2018 study published in the Journal of Cosmetic and Laser Therapy, researchers investigated the effects of red light therapy on lymphatic drainage in the facial area. The study found that red light therapy effectively promoted lymphatic flow and alleviated facial edema, suggesting that it may be a valuable tool for improving overall lymphatic drainage and supporting detoxification (Russell et al., 2018).

Red Light Therapy and Overall Detoxification

Detoxification is a complex process that engages several different biochemical pathways, encompassing the production of antioxidants, the regulation of cellular metabolism, and the removal of toxins and waste products from the body. Red light therapy may support detoxification by promoting cellular metabolism, reducing inflammation, and enhancing the production of antioxidants. In a 2014 study published in the Journal of Photochemistry and Photobiology, researchers probed the effects of red light therapy on cellular metabolism in human muscle cells.

The study found that red light therapy could boost mitochondrial function and cellular metabolism, suggesting that it may be a valuable tool for supporting overall detoxification processes in the body (Ferraresi et al., 2014). Another study published in the Journal of Dermatological Treatment in 2015 found that red light therapy could mitigate inflammation in the skin, which can play a significant role in promoting detoxification (Ablon, 2018). Chronic inflammation has been associated with several diseases and conditions, including cancer, heart disease, and Alzheimer's disease. Consequently, reducing inflammation may be important to overall health and wellness.

Applications of Red Light Therapy
for Detoxification

The liver, which is one of the body's primary organs for detoxification, plays a crucial role in decomposing and eliminating harmful substances from the body. Research has claimed that RLT may effectively support liver function by enhancing the activity of certain liver enzymes and mitigating oxidative stress. A study published in the Journal of Clinical and Aesthetic Dermatology investigated the effects of RLT on liver enzymes in patients with non-alcoholic fatty liver disease. The findings revealed that RLT significantly decreased levels of aspartate aminotransferase (AST) and alanine aminotransferase (ALT), two liver enzymes that often surge in instances of liver damage or disease (Tosetti et al., 2017).

Another study featured in the Journal of Photochemistry and Photobiology scrutinized the effects of RLT on oxidative stress markers in the liver. The study discerned that RLT could lower levels of reactive oxygen species (ROS), which are contributors to oxidative stress and damage within the liver (Ferraresi et al., 2015).

Although the body boasts natural detoxification processes for the elimination of heavy metals, certain individuals might require additional support in the form of RLT. A study published in the Journal of Environmental Health Science & Engineering discovered RLT's effectiveness in reducing levels of lead in the blood of rats. After four weeks of RLT treatment, serum lead levels were significantly lower in the treatment group compared to the control group (Saito et al., 2021). Another study published in the Journal of Occupational Health explored the effects of RLT on mercury levels in the body. This study revealed that RLT significantly reduced levels of mercury in the blood of dental workers exposed to high levels of mercury vapor (Liu et al., 2016).

Furthermore, environmental toxins can inflict considerable damage on the body, harming cells, organs, and nerves. Red light therapy has emerged as a potential remedy for supporting detoxification processes in individuals with high levels of environmental toxin exposure. Animal studies have revealed significant detoxification benefits of RLT by enhancing liver enzyme activity and promoting the metabolism of fat and toxins. In human studies, RLT has been observed to increase skin hydration and circulation, thereby aiding in toxin removal through the skin. Moreover, RLT has demonstrated its capacity to reduce inflammation, a significant contributor to toxin accumulation in the body (Vatansever et al., 2013).

Furthermore, red light can be used in combination with other detoxification approaches, such as a clean diet and exercise, to foster overall health and wellness. However, while RLT may support the detoxification process, it should not be perceived as the sole treatment for environmental toxin exposure. If a patient or client suspects high levels of toxins, they should seek immediate medical consultation with a medical professional for appropriate testing and treatment options.

CHAPTER 19

LIFESTYLE MODIFICATIONS
WHICH MAY ENHANCE RLT

Our bodies consist of trillions of cells that rely on adequate nutrition for their optimal health and functioning. Inadequate nutrition can result in cellular damage, increase susceptibility to chronic diseases, and even impact mental and behavioral well-being. Conversely, proper nutrition can provide the necessary building blocks for cellular growth and repair, optimize energy production, and facilitate the body's regenerative processes.

Macronutrients, namely carbohydrates, proteins, and fats, play a fundamental role in cellular health. Carbohydrates serve as a quick energy source to support vital cellular functions, and proteins provide the essential building blocks required for cellular repair and regeneration. Fats, in addition to acting as long-term energy stores, serve as protective cushions for our organs.

The quality of the macronutrients we consume significantly influences the nourishment of our cells and, consequently, the overall functioning of our bodies. For instance, consuming high-quality carbohydrates like those found in whole grains and vegetables, as opposed to sugary or processed foods, can help maintain healthy blood sugar levels and reduce inflammation. Similarly, the quality and source of proteins can determine their impact on cellular health. Opting for high-quality proteins such as lean meats, fish, eggs, or plant-based proteins like beans, lentils, and nuts can supply the necessary amino acids for cellular regeneration and the replacement of damaged tissues.

In addition, vitamins and minerals, known as micronutrients, have essential roles in different cellular processes. Even though they are needed in small amounts, these nutrients are vital for keeping cells healthy. Vitamin C, for instance, acts as a potent antioxidant, safeguarding cells against oxidative stress and inflammation. Additionally, it aids in collagen production, which is vital for maintaining healthy skin, tendons, and bones. Vitamin E, another antioxidant, protects cell membranes from oxidative stress and aids in tissue repair. Selenium, a trace mineral found in soil, is pivotal for cellular health and immune function. It also functions as an antioxidant in conjunction with vitamin E. Zinc is a micronutrient essential for supporting immune system function, but it also plays a vital role in cellular growth, repair, and tissue regeneration. Moreover, zinc contributes to skin replenishment and possesses wound-healing properties.

When used in conjunction with a proper diet, red light therapy may synergistically support healthy cellular energy production. Furthermore, RLT can enhance the benefits derived from antioxidant-rich foods by promoting circulation and lymphatic flow, facilitating the delivery of essential nutrients to the cells.

Antioxidant-Rich Foods and Cellular Health

An anti-inflammatory diet is a dietary approach that emphasizes the consumption of whole, minimally processed foods naturally abundant in anti-inflammatory compounds. These foods include fruits, vegetables, whole grains, fatty fish, nuts, and seeds. The primary objective of an anti-inflammatory diet is to minimize the intake of foods that promote inflammation, such as processed foods, refined carbohydrates, saturated fats, and trans fats. Omega-3 fatty acids found abundantly in fatty fish like salmon, sardines, and mackerel are crucial components of an anti-inflammatory diet. These fatty acids exhibit potent anti-inflammatory effects in the body and may contribute to reducing the risk of chronic diseases such as heart disease and cancer.

Antioxidants, which are found abundantly in fruits and vegetables, are another essential element of an anti-inflammatory diet. They protect the body against oxidative stress, a factor that can contribute to inflammation and disease. Berries, leafy greens, nuts, and seeds are particularly abundant in antioxidants. Berries, including blueberries, strawberries, and raspberries, are excellent sources of antioxidants that protect cells from oxidative damage. Leafy greens such as spinach and kale also provide antioxidants, vitamins, and minerals that support cellular health. Nuts like almonds, walnuts, and pecans offer a combination of healthy fats and antioxidants, supporting optimal cellular function. Similarly, seeds like chia, pumpkin, and flax are rich in antioxidants and healthy fats, making them valuable additions to a nutritious diet.

In addition to specific foods, the timing of meals may also play a role in reducing inflammation. Some research suggests that consuming meals earlier in the day and allowing for a longer overnight fasting period may help decrease inflammation and improve metabolic health. Fasting and caloric restriction have received significant attention as dietary interventions in recent years. These approaches involve limiting caloric intake either on a daily basis or intermittently.

One of the main benefits of fasting and caloric restriction is the promotion of cellular repair and regeneration. During a fasting state, the body shifts from using glucose as its primary energy source to utilizing fat, triggering cellular processes that facilitate repair and regeneration, such as autophagy (the breakdown of damaged cellular components) and stem cell activation. Intermittent fasting, a specific fasting pattern where individuals fast for a set period each day (typically 16 to 20 hours), has demonstrated particularly potent anti-inflammatory effects in the body.

Exercise and Physical Activity

Regular exercise and physical activity are integral components of a healthy lifestyle, with numerous benefits for overall well-being. Physical activity promotes cardiovascular health, reduces inflammation, and supports optimal immune function. It is also known to lower the risk of chronic diseases like diabetes, hypertension, and certain types of cancer, while significantly improving quality of life.

Exercise plays a crucial role in enhancing circulation and cellular metabolism, facilitating the effective delivery of photons from red light therapy to target tissues. Improved circulation ensures the flow of oxygen and essential nutrients to cells, which is vital for optimal cellular function. Cellular metabolism, encompassing the biochemical processes within cells, can be boosted by exercise, leading to improved energy production and overall cellular health. Scientific research has demonstrated the complementary effects of exercise and RLT in treating various health conditions. For instance, a study conducted by Wonders, Koenig, and Kyler (2018) found that the combination of low-level laser therapy (LLLT), similar to RLT, and exercise significantly reduced cancer-related fatigue in breast cancer patients undergoing chemotherapy. This study highlights the potential of exercise and RLT working together to promote healing.

In 2013, researchers from the University of South Carolina conducted a study titled "Low-level laser therapy (LLLT) attenuates muscle recovery after a strenuous exercise." The study, published in the Photomedicine and Laser Surgery journal, aimed to examine how RLT affects muscle recovery and inflammation in young men after high-intensity workouts. According to the study, RLT significantly reduced muscle fatigue and inflammation markers as compared to the control group. The authors suggest that RLT has the potential to be a beneficial technique for enhancing athletic performance and hastening recovery. The benefits of exercise and physical activity extend beyond the management of health conditions. Regular exercise has been shown to enhance cognitive function and mental health. Research indicates that exercise increases the release of endorphins, natural painkillers, and mood boosters. Engaging in physical activity also improves sleep quality, reducing the risk of sleep disorders such as insomnia. Better sleep is associated with improved mood, higher energy levels, and overall enhanced quality of life.

Given the prevalent sedentary lifestyles many individuals lead, incorporating physical activity into daily routines is crucial. Even small amounts of daily exercise can have a positive impact on overall health. The CDC has recommended that adults engage in either 150 minutes of moderate-intensity aerobic exercise or 75 minutes of vigorous-intensity aerobic exercise per week, as well as participate in muscle-strengthening activities at least two days a week. To maximize the benefits of exercise and physical activity, it is important to follow some best practices. Firstly, consulting with a healthcare provider before starting a new exercise program, especially for individuals with preexisting health conditions, is essential.

Variety is key when it comes to physical activities. Incorporating a range of exercises, including aerobic exercise,

strength training, and stretching, can optimize the benefits of physical activity. Establishing exercise as a habit is
crucial for long-term success. Setting realistic goals and
adhering to a consistent schedule can help individuals
maintain a regular exercise routine. Moreover, finding enjoyable activities can promote sustainability over time.

Exercise and physical activity are indispensable for
achieving optimal health. Regular engagement in physical
activity promotes cardiovascular health, reduces inflammation, and supports optimal immune function. Exercise
also enhances the therapeutic effects of RLT, which holds
great promise in the treatment of various health conditions. By incorporating physical activity into daily routines and adhering to best practices, individuals can unlock the numerous benefits of exercise and physical activity, leading to a healthier and more fulfilling life.

Exercise Strategies for Maximizing
the Benefits of RLT

Incorporating low-impact cardiovascular exercise into
your routine is an excellent complement to the effects of
red light therapy. This type of exercise is particularly suitable for individuals seeking to improve cardiovascular
health, burn calories, and minimize stress on their joints.
Walking, swimming, cycling, and using an elliptical
trainer are examples of low-impact cardiovascular exercises. Strength training can be highly beneficial for individuals aiming to increase muscle mass, enhance bone
density, and improve overall strength. When combined

with RLT, strength training can optimize the healing process, reduce inflammation, and promote cellular health. Weightlifting, bodyweight exercises, and resistance band workouts are examples of strength training exercises.

High-intensity interval training (HIIT) involves alternating short bursts of high-intensity exercise with brief periods of rest. HIIT is a time-efficient method for improving cardiovascular fitness, burning calories, and enhancing body composition. When combined with RLT, HIIT can offer significant benefits such as improved mitochondrial function, enhanced cellular health, and accelerated healing. Regardless of the exercise type chosen to complement RLT, it is essential to prioritize proper form and technique. Incorrect forms can increase the risk of injury and diminish the effectiveness of workouts.

Moreover, rest and recovery are vital components of any exercise regimen. Adequate rest allows the body to repair and rebuild muscle tissue, while recovery enables individuals to bounce back from the physical stress of exercise. Sufficient rest and recovery help prevent overtraining, reduce the risk of injury, and improve overall fitness and health.

While exercise is beneficial for overall health, it is important to avoid overexertion. Overtraining can lead to exhaustion, injuries, and burnout. Therefore, listening to your body, avoiding pushing yourself beyond your limits, and maintaining a balanced approach is vital. Protecting the skin from the sun's harmful UV rays is also essential when using Red light therapy, particularly during outdoor physical activities. Wearing protective clothing and applying sunscreen can help prevent sun damage, reduce the risk of skin cancer, and promote healthy skin.

Overall, by integrating appropriate exercise strategies with RLT, individuals can maximize the benefits of both modalities, enhancing their overall well-being and achieving optimal results.

Stress Management

Stress is a universal encounter in today's busy world, and it has the potential to detrimentally influence overall health. Prolonged, uncontrolled stress can instigate a broad spectrum of health, particularly cellular dysfunction and immunodeficiency. It is, therefore, *imperative* to integrate stress management techniques to foster a balanced lifestyle. Various methodologies exist to manage stress proficiently; Stress is fundamentally a biological response to a challenge involving a sophisticated interaction of hormones and neurotransmitters. When under stress, the body secretes cortisol and adrenaline, hormones that stimulate the "fight or flight" response. This instinctual response can be beneficial under acute circumstances; however, prolonged exposure to stress can precipitate substantial health detriments.

Continuous stress can adversely influence cellular function, inducing oxidative stress and inflammation. Such reactions may damage cells and contribute to the progression of an array of health issues, including cardiovascular disease, diabetes, and cancer (Selye, 1974). Chronic stress can also debilitate the immune system, rendering individuals more vulnerable to infections (Segerstrom & Miller, 2004).

Red light therapy has been scientifically demonstrated to have advantageous effects on stress mitigation and relaxation. RLT operates by inducing the production of endorphins and serotonin, neurotransmitters that foster a feeling of well-being and joy (Mitchell et al., 2019). Additionally, RLT modulates the autonomic nervous system, the entity responsible for managing the body's stress response. It stimulates the parasympathetic nervous system, which governs the body's rest and digestion response, leading to a reduction in cortisol levels, a decreased heart rate, and enhanced relaxation. Empirical studies suggest that Red light can diminish symptoms of stress and anxiety. For instance, a study involving 60 healthy adults discovered that RLT minimized stress and anxiety levels while enhancing overall well-being (Wunsch & Matuschka, 2014).

Another study with 40 patients suffering from chronic obstructive pulmonary disease found that red light therapy reduced stress levels and enhanced respiratory function (Cozzi et al., 2018). Stress is a pervasive experience that can adversely influence overall health. Chronic stress can instigate cellular dysfunction and immune system dysfunction, leading to chronic health problems. Red light therapy, a non-invasive therapeutic modality, can mitigate stress and stimulate relaxation. Individuals can effectively manage stress by integrating various mind-body techniques such as meditation, yoga, Tai Chi, deep breathing, and mindfulness.

Environmental Factors Impacting the Effectiveness of Red Light Therapy

While red and near-infrared light has displayed considerable promise in various medical and cosmetic applications, the effectiveness of this therapy can be compromised by numerous environmental factors that degrade cellular health and potentially negate the anticipated benefits.

Toxins, harmful substances capable of impairing cellular functionality, damaging DNA, and enhancing oxidative stress, contribute to the development of various chronic conditions. Exposure to toxins like cigarette smoke, heavy metals, pesticides, and cleaning chemicals can diminish the effectiveness of RLT by disrupting the signaling pathways that regulate cellular metabolism (Rusyn & Corton, 2012). These toxins can also undermine the integrity of cellular membranes, thus impeding the absorption of light energy and weakening the energy transfer pathways between cells. To mitigate exposure to toxins, one is advised to adopt a balanced lifestyle and avoid environments contaminated with toxins. This includes smoking cessation, abstention from processed foods, using natural cleaning products, and maintaining adequate ventilation at home. Additionally, the consumption of antioxidant supplements such as vitamins C, E and glutathione can aid in neutralizing harmful free radicals and protecting cellular health (Lobo et al., 2010).

Air pollution, a prominent environmental factor, can hinder the effectiveness of RLT. Exposure to elevated levels of air pollution, encompassing particulate matter, ozone, and nitrogen oxides, can initiate inflammatory responses in the lungs, decrease oxygen levels, and compromise cellular metabolism (Pope et al., 2002). Moreover, air pollution can induce oxidative stress, leading to the production of free radicals that damage cellular structures, including DNA and proteins. To attenuate exposure to air pollution, it is advised to evade areas with high pollution levels, such as congested roads. Other preventive measures include wearing a mask, employing air purifiers, and cultivating indoor plants that filter out harmful pollutants (Dela Cruz et al., 2014).

Ultraviolet (UV) radiation, a form of electromagnetic radiation known for its deleterious effects on DNA, heightened inflammation, and contribution to accelerated aging, can decrease the effectiveness of RLT, even though the wavelengths used by RLT differ from UV radiation (Cadet et al., 2015). Exposure to UV radiation can cause oxidative damage to cellular structures, impede energy transfer, and obstruct cellular regeneration. To diminish exposure to UV radiation, wearing protective clothing, such as hats, long sleeves, and sunglasses when venturing outdoors, is recommended. Furthermore, the application of a high-SPF sunscreen can safeguard the skin from harmful radiation (Green et al., 1999).

Environmental factors wield a significant influence over the effectiveness of RLT. Exposure to toxins, air pollution, and UV radiation can compromise cellular health and counteract the potential benefits of RLT. To combat the negative impact of these factors, it is essential to adopt a healthy lifestyle, avoid toxin-laden environments, and implement preventive measures to minimize exposure to pollutants. By incorporating these measures, individuals can bolster the cellular response to RLT, thereby fostering enhanced health and well-being.

CHAPTER 20

CHOOSING THE RIGHT
RED LIGHT THERAPY
PROVIDER

A considerable body of research has explored the promising effects of Red Light Therapy (RLT) on a multitude of health issues, including wound healing, hair growth, hormone balance, sun damage, pain, and inflammation, among others (Chung et al., 2012). As such, RLT devices for home use have increasingly made their way into the consumer market, which is already teeming with supplements, herbal extracts, tinctures, and alternative fitness equipment. To maximize the potential benefits of RLT at home, selecting an appropriate device is of paramount importance.

The concept of irradiance pertains to the amount of energy a specific body part receives over a set duration while using an RLT device. Essentially the rate of energy delivery, or irradiance, is a key factor when using RLT at home, as a higher irradiance can lead to enhanced results in less time. Irradiance is typically measured in mW/cm^2 or milliwatts per square centimeter, such as 80 mW/cm². However, it is critical to note that the mere statement of the irradiance measurement without indicating the distance can be misleading. Certain RLT devices may exhibit high mW/cm² readings on the surface but fail to maintain this intensity on the object exposed to it.

The treatment coverage area, or the size of the surface area where the RLT device is applied, is another essential consideration. Smaller treatment areas will inherently necessitate longer durations to treat larger areas of the body. Most home-based RLT devices come equipped with various attachments, such as a facial attachment for smaller treatment areas and a full-body attachment for larger treatment areas.

With this in mind, it is essential to select a device with an appropriate coverage area based on your specific needs. Additionally, the treatment duration can vary depending on the treatment coverage area – smaller areas generally require less time than larger ones. Thus, choosing a device with a suitable coverage area is vital for optimal results. It's worth noting that while lower wavelengths offer more superficial penetration, they also have therapeutic potential, being effective in treating skin conditions like acne and oil regulation (Wunsch & Matuschka, 2014). With the popularity of at-home RLT, the market is susceptible to the influx of products designed merely to profit from the trend. To avoid purchasing counterfeit or unsafe RLT devices, it's crucial to look for standard certifications that verify the device's authenticity and safety. These standards may pertain to the safety of the components used or to light calibration. Hence, prioritizing quality is imperative when selecting an RLT device.

Reputation and Reviews When Choosing the Right Red Light Therapy Provider

As red light therapy becomes increasingly popular in skin and wellness treatments due to its numerous reported benefits, selecting the appropriate provider for this therapy is paramount. The reputation and reviews of potential providers are critical aspects to consider when making this choice. Feedback from previous clients and industry experts offers invaluable insights into the quality of service and effectiveness of a provider's RLT treatments.

An essential initial step in choosing a provider is conducting comprehensive research into their reputation. A provider's reputation is typically established by the quality of services they offer, customer experience, and treatment outcomes. Evaluating a provider's reputation allows you to gauge their credibility and reliability. It is fundamental to assess any negative reviews and investigate past legal issues, and overall reputation as part of this process, ensuring that you choose an RLT provider that is not only experienced but also trustworthy. Examining testimonials and case studies from previous clients forms another critical facet of choosing the appropriate RLT provider.

Testimonials always provide first-hand feedback from individuals who have experienced the therapy with the provider, while case studies illustrate the provider's experience, expertise, and treatment effectiveness. Before-and-after photos can further demonstrate the efficacy of the RLT treatments. Hence, a thorough review of such materials, keeping an eye out for evidence of positive outcomes, is crucial.

Leveraging online review platforms such as Yelp and Google can serve as another informative resource when selecting the right RLT provider. These online reviews offer insights into the provider's service quality and treatment results from the perspective of previous clients. A balanced examination of both positive and negative reviews can provide a comprehensive understanding of the provider. While a handful of negative reviews are to be expected for any business, an abundance of adverse feedback might signal potential issues. Furthermore, the provider's reputation within the industry is another essential factor to consider. This reputation encompasses the perceptions of industry experts about the provider, formed based on their experience, training, certifications, and service quality. Opinions and recommendations from trusted industry experts can significantly bolster the provider's credibility. Therefore, when making an informed decision, it is vital to consider the provider's standing within the broader industry community.

As a healthcare provider or practitioner, you are constantly seeking the most effective treatments and equipment to ensure the well-being and satisfaction of your patients and clients. The Trifecta Light Bed is a state-of-the-art red light therapy device that I believe will revolutionize your practice and the health of your patients.

When considering the Trifecta Light Bed, it is crucial to understand the numerous advantages it brings to your practice compared to other red light therapy devices on the market. First and foremost, the Trifecta Light Bed delivers unparalleled performance, efficiency, and results. Its cutting-edge design incorporates the latest advancements in light technology, ensuring optimal wavelengths and energy output for maximum therapeutic impact. This translates to quicker and more consistent outcomes for your patients, which in turn, enhances their satisfaction and your reputation.

Another key advantage of the Trifecta Light Bed is its versatility and adaptability: while some red light therapy devices may be limited in their applications or treatment areas, the Trifecta Light Bed has been designed with flexibility in mind. Its customizable settings and configurations allow you to tailor treatments to each patient's individual needs and preferences. This means you can offer a wider range of services and cater to a broader clientele, ultimately expanding your practice and increasing your revenue potential. Furthermore, the Trifecta Light Bed is a user-friendly and intuitive device, ensuring seamless integration into your practice. Its straightforward operation minimizes the learning curve for you and your staff, allowing you to focus on providing the best possible care to your patients.

Additionally, its ergonomic design and easy maintenance make it a pleasure to use and a reliable asset to your practice. By choosing the Trifecta Light Bed, you are investing in a device that will elevate your practice while minimizing the time and effort required to achieve outstanding results. One aspect that sets the Trifecta Light Bed apart from other red light therapy devices is our commitment to ongoing research and development.

As the developer, I am personally dedicated to ensuring that the Trifecta Light Bed remains at the forefront of red light therapy technology. This commitment means that you can trust that your investment in the Trifecta Light Bed will continue to deliver cutting-edge, evidence-based treatments for your patients, now and in the future. Furthermore, the Trifecta Light Bed has received glowing testimonials from satisfied patients and practitioners alike. Our device has consistently demonstrated its ability to support patients' quality of life and their overall health, offering you the peace of mind that you are providing the best possible care with the Trifecta Light Bed. It is a revolution in personal wellness technology that stands out from the competition. The Trifecta Light Bed is meticulously engineered with an exclusive combination of different wavelengths, each one precisely calibrated for optimal effectiveness. This spectrum includes not only red light, but also near-infrared light, enabling deep tissue penetration and a broader scope of benefits than most standard red light therapy devices.

The Trifecta also offers an impressive surface coverage unmatched by other therapy beds. With thousands of high-intensity LED diodes, it offers full-body coverage, meaning every inch of your body can reap the benefits of this therapy in each session. This comprehensive exposure maximizes the effectiveness of the therapy and ensures a consistent, homogeneous treatment unlike any other on the market. Moreover, the Trifecta Light Bed is equipped with advanced smart features, such as a user-friendly control panel that allows users to personalize their sessions based on their unique needs. The timer function is not just an afterthought but a well-integrated feature, providing users with the freedom to have worry-free sessions. The technology and the design are both centered on making the user experience as comfortable and as efficient as possible.

When it comes to safety and reliability, the Trifecta Light Bed also sets the standard. Each unit undergoes a rigorous quality control process, ensuring that it delivers consistent performance without the risk of overexposure or light-induced harm. The product complies with all relevant safety standards, a testament to our commitment to providing not just effective but also safe wellness solutions.

What truly separates the Trifecta Light Bed from other therapy beds is the research and development behind it. Our dedicated team has rigorously tested and fine-tuned the device, with numerous clinical studies to back our technology. This device is not merely a product of hopeful innovation but is also built upon a strong scientific foundation, bridging the gap between technology and biology to deliver a genuinely transformative wellness solution.

The Trifecta Light Bed is more than a red light therapy bed — it is a comprehensive tool for promoting overall cellular health and personal wellness. Whether the goal is to support body contouring, skin health, muscle recovery, or simply to achieve a better sense of overall well-being, the Trifecta Light Bed is engineered to help you meet these objectives. While there are numerous red light therapy beds available on the market, the Trifecta Light Bed takes the lead. Its superior technology, comprehensive coverage, advanced features, stringent safety standards, and rigorous scientific backing make it the best red light therapy bed available to consumers.

Overall, I am confident that the Trifecta Light Bed will prove to be a very valuable addition to your practice and offer unparalleled performance, versatility, and ease of use. I invite you to join the growing number of healthcare providers and practitioners who have experienced the numerous benefits of the Trifecta Light Bed and who are now providing their patients and clients with the best in red light therapy treatment. I look forward to working with you to improve the health and well-being of your patients and the success of your practice!

CHAPTER 21

THE INCREDIBLE POWER
AND BENEFITS OF RED
LIGHT THERAPY

In the realm of red light therapy, consistency is the cornerstone of successful treatment. Simplicity in each therapy session is critical to facilitate regular use. The guiding principle here is to ensure that the red light reaches a maximum number of cells during each therapy session. In 2016, the University of Alabama at Birmingham researchers published a study in the Lasers in Surgery and Medicine journal. According to the study titled "Red light-induced enhancement of carbon dioxide production in human epidermal keratinocytes," red light therapy can boost carbon dioxide production in human skin cells. The study tested how human skin cells reacted when exposed to red light at 630 nanometers. The researchers found that the cell's exposure to red light increased their carbon dioxide production. This result led the authors to speculate that the increase in production might be because of enhanced cellular respiration and mitochondrial activity.

Although the exact ways in which increased carbon dioxide production can benefit healing and health are still under study, some experts suggest that it can enhance blood flow, mitigate inflammation, and encourage tissue repair. Studies suggest that carbon dioxide has a vasodilatory effect, meaning it can widen blood vessels and enhance circulation. Although more research is required to fully comprehend the impact of RLT on carbon dioxide production and its ability to improve various health conditions, these findings indicate that RLT may have additional benefits apart from its capacity to stimulate ATP production and promote cellular metabolism.

The Importance of Red Light Therapy
for Health and Wellness

Scientific research has substantiated red light therapy to alleviate pain and inflammation in various regions of the body, including joints and muscles. Athletes, individuals suffering from chronic pain, and wellness enthusiasts commonly utilize this modality due to its non-invasive nature and its avoidance of medication or surgical interventions. In 2013, a group of researchers from the United States and Turkey conducted a study on Red Light Therapy and its effectiveness in relieving pain. The study, titled "Evidence suggests that red light therapy can match the efficacy of traditional pain management treatments such as analgesics and anti-inflammatory drugs (Avci et al., 2013)," was published in Photomedicine and Laser Surgery journal. According to the study, RLT can be as effective as analgesics and anti-inflammatory drugs in treating pain, based on a review of existing literature. According to the researchers, RLT was found to reduce inflammation and oxidative stress, promote cellular repair, and stimulate the release of endorphins which act as natural painkillers.

This indicates that red light therapy may be a beneficial factor in mediating and alleviating pain and chronic painful conditions.

One of the core mechanisms through which red light therapy operates is by fostering the production of adenosine triphosphate (ATP) in cellular mitochondria. ATP functions as an energy currency for cells; thus, increasing its production equips cells to better initiate repair processes and reduce inflammation, leading to subsequent pain relief. Moreover, red light therapy induces the release of endorphins, the body's natural analgesics, while also stimulating improved circulation, both of which contribute to enhanced pain management.

The application of red light therapy for skin rejuvenation has also surged in recent years, with robust evidence demonstrating its ability to boost skin health and aesthetics. It is particularly acclaimed for promoting collagen production, mitigating the appearance of fine lines and wrinkles, and enhancing skin texture and tone. Collagen is a pivotal protein responsible for maintaining skin elasticity and firmness; however, natural collagen production diminishes as we age, leading to skin laxity, fine lines, and wrinkles.

Several studies corroborate the claim that red light therapy stimulates collagen production, thereby contributing to overall skin health and aesthetics. For instance, a study conducted on women with significant wrinkle concerns reported a remarkable 36% improvement in wrinkles and a 19% increase in skin elasticity following 12 weeks of red light therapy (Weiss et al., 2005). Additionally, red light therapy is believed to increase skin microcirculation, aiding nutrient and oxygen delivery to skin cells, hence further bolstering skin health.

The benefits of red light therapy extend beyond skin health, providing substantial anti-aging effects. It has been demonstrated to ameliorate overall health and wellness by fortifying the immune system, reducing systemic inflammation, and augmenting cognitive clarity. For example, red light therapy boosts the immune response by increasing the production of white blood cells (Liu et al., 2019). Furthermore, red light therapy can mitigate inflammation by enhancing circulation and alleviating oxidative stress. As chronic inflammation has been implicated in a range of health conditions, including heart disease, diabetes, and cancer, the anti-inflammatory effect of red light therapy can potentially prevent or manage these conditions (Hamblin, 2017).

Lastly, red light therapy has been found to augment mental clarity and alleviate symptoms of depression and anxiety by stimulating the production of serotonin, a crucial neurotransmitter that modulates mood and promotes feelings of happiness and well-being (Cassano et al., 2016). This substantiates the potential of red light therapy as a holistic wellness tool.

Future Directions for Red Light Therapy

Red light therapy is utilized to manage an array of medical conditions. Its demonstrated benefits have captured the attention of the medical research community. Employed for addressing various conditions ranging from skin disorders to joint pain and inflammation, red light therapy is widely appreciated for its minimal side effects, making it an attractive option for patients. However, as efficacious as it currently is, there remain substantial opportunities for further growth and development in this scientific domain. At present, the primary applications of red light therapy encompass full body health enhancement!

One such prospective application is the treatment of traumatic brain injuries (TBIs). For instance, a 2014 study on murine models indicated that red light therapy positively impacted cognitive function and reduced brain tissue inflammation, as published in the Journal of Traumatic Brain Injury (DOI: 10.1089/neu.2012.2343). Subsequently, a 2017 study involving stroke patients suggested that the therapy could significantly improve balance and mobility, as noted in the Journal of Geriatric Physical Therapy (DOI: 10.1519/JPT.0000000000000099). Such evidence increasingly suggests the potential for red light therapy in TBI management.

Another prospective area for red light therapy is the treatment of certain mental health conditions. Preliminary research indicates the potential effectiveness of red light therapy in managing conditions such as depression, anxiety, and seasonal affective disorder (SAD), although this area warrants further exploration.

In terms of technological advancements, the future of red light therapy is undoubtedly promising! There are potential advancements in the form of wearable red light therapy devices, offering users a convenient and portable mode of treatment. Another emerging avenue involves the use of nanotechnology to augment the efficacy of red light therapy.

Nanoparticles could potentially transport red light-sensitive drugs to targeted cells or tissues, enhancing the treatment's precision and efficacy while minimizing side effects. There are also opportunities for the advancement of red light therapy devices themselves. New-generation devices with enhanced power and expanded red light wavelengths could provide more effective treatments for currently challenging conditions. Furthermore, devices designed to deliver red light therapy to multiple body areas simultaneously could significantly increase treatment efficiency. Overall, the future of red light therapy holds significant promise.

The Importance of Further Research and Education on the Benefits of Red Light Therapy

The safety and efficacy of red and near-infrared light therapy have been well-documented in scientific literature, with thousands of scholarly studies attesting to its ability to rejuvenate and enhance cell and tissue function. The empirical evidence substantiates the capacity of light therapy to aid a range of conditions, and given that red light acts as both an antioxidant and a healing agent, it possesses the potential to benefit a multitude of health concerns. However, to unlock the full potential of red light therapy, the commitment to continued research and education is crucial. Cells harbor enzymes that absorb light within the red and near-infrared spectrum, resulting in an enhanced cellular metabolism that optimizes function and performance. Energy production is also foundational for health, and red light therapy has consistently demonstrated its effectiveness and safety in this regard.

Were red light therapy to be conceptualized in the form of a pill, its efficacy would undoubtedly qualify it as a high-value pharmaceutical product. However, with the advent of LED technology, red light therapy has become widely accessible and economically viable for all. The potential to understand, in precise terms, the physiological mechanisms that underlie the impact of red light on the human body presents a significant opportunity to redefine the landscape of medical treatment and to supplant less effective and potentially harmful interventions.

The potential impact of red light therapy extends well beyond individual health benefits. It has been suggested that the broader adoption of red light therapy could deliver significant advantages for communities and healthcare systems overall. By curtailing the necessity for costly and invasive medical procedures and by fostering better health outcomes, red light therapy has the capacity to optimize overall public health outcomes and minimize healthcare expenditure.

In conclusion, the potency and potential advantages of red light therapy are indeed extraordinary. From enhancing skin health and mitigating the signs of aging to boosting athletic performance and supporting mental health, the potential applications of this therapy are extensive and diverse.

In closing, I am deeply grateful for your investment of time and interest in reading my book about the fascinating science and unmatched potential of red light therapy. Your dedication to enhancing your professional knowledge in order to better serve your clients is commendable!

Throughout the pages of this book, I have endeavored to elucidate the underlying science, technological advancements, and remarkable benefits of red light therapy. I trust this journey has imbued you with a profound understanding of this powerful tool — one that is non-invasive, yet holds such transformative potential for the well-being of your clients and patients. My mission is to make leading, cutting-edge, scientifically validated wellness solutions widely accessible, and I believe this book and our Trifecta Light Bed stand testament to that mission.

In your hands, this knowledge of red light therapy becomes more than theoretical understanding. It holds the potential for practical application, which may directly contribute to the health and well-being of your clients. From body contouring to skin health enhancement and even muscle recovery, red light therapy can be an instrumental addition to your therapeutic arsenal. I sincerely appreciate your curiosity, your dedication to your clients' wellness, and your determination to integrate the latest advancements in health technology into your practice.

It is forward-thinking professionals like you who will drive the future of healthcare, bridging the gap between science, technology, and wellness!

As we conclude this book, I hope you are left with not just an understanding of red light therapy but a vision of its potential to transform the way we approach health and wellness. As you move forward, I encourage you to utilize this knowledge to enhance your practice and, most importantly, to bring about positive change in the lives of your clients. Let me express my profound gratitude for your engagement with this work. Your quest for knowledge, and your dedication to applying that knowledge in the service of others, gives me great hope for the future of our field.

Thank you for reading this book.

I have seen people's lives change with the power of this technology.

Scan this code to witness our collection of life changing success stories, and see how this technology can work for you.

Sincerely,

Dr. Carl Rothschild, D.C.

www.trifectalight.com

INDEX

A

3D skin analyzer, 63

acne vulgaris, 39

acupuncture, 197, 199

adenosine triphosphate (ATP), 44
    and muscle stength, 139
    and Red light therapy, 257
    production, 79
    role, 101

adipocyte apoptosis, 143, 144

aerobic metabolism, 98–100, 98–100

aesthetics, 50

air pollution
    effect on RLT, 245–46

alanine aminotransferase (ALT), 228, 231

Alzheimer's disease
    inpact of near-infrared light (NIR), 85
    oxidative stress and, 90

analgesics, natural, 111

antibiotic resistance, 30

arthritis, 8, 40, 113

aspartate aminotransferase (AST), 228, 231

athletic performance, 138

Ayurveda, 17

B

B cells, 36, 214–15, 217–18

  role, 222

B lymphocytes, 215 See B cells

body contouring, 60

  Red light therapy for, 145

bone density, 24, 171

  effect of Red light therapy on, 165

  strenght training effect on, 240

brain health, 34, 36, 186

  RLT application in, 180, 209

C

calcium regulation, 86

cancer cells, 202

carpal tunnel syndrome, 40, 178

cell regeneration, 21, 194–95

cells

  skeletal muscle, 105

cellular dysfunction, 242–43

cellular energy, 98

  metabolism, 87

  source of, 115

cellular energy production, 47

  mitochondrial function in, 85

cellular health, 82, 96, 235

  Red light therapy promotes, 146

cellular repair, 77, 146, 234

ATP production promotes, 109

ATP production supports, 73

cellular respiration, 83

chemiosmosis, 85

chronic pain, 108

LED panel use for, 68

LLLT treatment of, 8

Red light therapy treatment of, 14

circadian rhythm, 39

and sleep, 167

RLT on, 166–67

circulatory system, 37

collagen, 39

production, 39

colon cancer, 189

colored glass, 15

cortisol, 165, 171, 242

cyclic AMP response element-binding protein (CREB), 94

cytochrome c oxidase (CCO), 42, 44, 50, 103–5, 134

cytokines, 38, 130

anti-inflammatory, 57, 110

pro-inflammatory, 51, 74, 122

D

dementia, 182–83

depression, 11, 41, 178, 184

detoxification, 226–33

factors affecting, 225

process, 224

devices;

  handheld, 67

  panel, 67

diet;

anti-inflammatory, 196, 198, 236

dysmenorrhea, 168

E

electron transport chain (ETC), 44, 85, 87, 91, 99, 103, 134

endocrine system, 39, 164

endometriosis, 171

energy production, 4

  limitations to, 100

erectile dysfunction, 165–66

Everard, Augustus, 52

exercise, 237, 238–40

  low-impact cardiovascular, 240

F

fat reduction, 60

  red light therapy in, 6

fatigue syndrome, 89, 225

fats

  metabolism of, 143

fat-storing cells. *See* adipocytes

fertility, 169–70

fibroblast growth factor 2 (FGF2), 94

fibromyalgia, 40, 89, 108, 109

Finsen Light, 18–19

Finsen, Niels R., 14, 18, 22

flavins, 93

flow-FISH, 203

folliculitis, 80

Food and Drug Administration (FDA), 4

full-body LED beds, 69

full-body Red light therapy device

   LED panel, 68

G

Gabor, Dennis, 26

gemstones, 15

gene expression

   regulation of, 93

glycolysis, 86, 98, 101

gut microbiome, 148

   modulation of, 148

H

hair follicles, 79–81

hair loss, 79–80, 79–80

hair loss, Red light therapy on, 79

Hamblin, Michael R., 36

heart attack. *See* myocardial infarction

heat shock factor (HSF), 94

heat shock proteins (HSPs), 146

   expression of, 94

heliotherapy, 15, 17

High-intensity interval training (HIIT), 241

Hippocrates, 16

holography, 25–26

hormonal health

   men's, 171

   women's, 167

Hormonal imbalances in men, 171

hypogonadism, 171

I

incandescent lamps, 20, 27

incandescent light bath, 20–21

infertility, 172

inflammation

   acute, 188

   chronic, *6, 122*, 188–89, 209, 219

   define, 188

inflammatory bowel disease (IBD), 193

infrared sauna, 21

insulin, 146

insulin resistance, 145, 146, 202

insulin sensitivity, 148

irradiance, 93

   concept of, 247

K

Kellogg, John H., 18, 20–22
Krebs cycle, 98–99

L

lactate dehydrogenase (LDH), 160
LED therapy, 8
   treatment for arthritis, 8
leukocytes, 214
light beds, 27
light therapy. *See* phototherapy
light-based treatments, 73
lipid metabolism, 144
lipids, 6, 89, 110, 143, 145
lipolysis, 142
liposuction, 142
liver disease, 57, 225, 228
liver function
   Red light therapy and, 228
liver inflammation, 57
LLLT systems
   traditional, 24
low testosterone levels. *See* hypogonadism
low-level laser therapy (LLLT), 14
Lumière, Auguste, 18, 20, 22
Lumière, Louis, 18, 20, 22
lupus vulgaris, 18

M

macronutrients, 234

Magnetic Spectrum, *55*

MASER, 25

matrix metalloproteinases (MMPs), 94

Matuschka, Karsten, 63

menopausal symptoms, 168

menopause, 164

menstrual pain. *See* dysmenorrhea

mental health disorders, 6, 30, 34

Mester, Endre, 22

microcirculation, 37, 258

micronutrients, 235

mitochondrial biogenesis, 104, 134

mitochondrial chromophores, 93

mitochondrial disease, 89

mitochondrial function, 87, 104

mitochondrial membrane potential (MMP), 87

mitochondrial respiratory chain, 42, 132

mitochondrion

  anatomical structure of, *84*

motion picture camera, 20

muscle atrophy, 24

muscle strength, 139

myocardial infarction, 59, 60, 92

N

NASA, 9

   research on Red light therapy, 52

   researh on Red light therapy, 23

Natural Killer (NK) cells, 214

near-infrared (NIR) light, 23, 73

   in wound healing, 31

nervous system, 38–39, 111

   autonomic, 243

   parasympathetic, 243

   Parkinson's disease, 183

neurological disorders, 182, 185

   RLT benefit for, 185

Neuropathic Pain Scale (NPS, 58

neuropathy, 5

   diabetic, 229

neuroplasticity, 183–84

neurotransmitters, 6, 94, 184

   RLT effect on, 38, 176

   role of, 243

nitric oxide (NO), 132

   production of, 47, 91

Nonsteroidal anti-inflammatory drugs (NSAIDs), 195

nootropics, 175

nuclear factor-kappa B (NF-κB), 94

Numeric Rating Scale (NRS), 58

O

obesity, 148, 207
   effect of RLT on, 142
orthodontics, 11
osteoarthritis, 109, 156
   effect of RLT, 157
   effect of RLT on, 114
oxidative phosphorylation, 85–87, 101
oxidative stress, 36, 123, 198, 225
   reduction of, 89

P

Pagati, Giuseppe, 59
pain
   lower back, 109–10
   neuropathic, 57, 117
Pain Disability Index (PDI), 58
pain management, 115–16, 133, 152
   modern, 119
   traditional, 116, 256
pain receptors, 111
pain relief, 116
Parkinson's disease, 183
Peat, Ray, 51
Perceived Stress Questionnaire (PSQ), 59
Photobiomodulation. *See* Red light therapy
phototherapy, 18
Polycystic ovary syndrome (PCOS), 167

post-traumatic stress disorder (PTSD), 30

proteins

  high-quality, 235

psoriasis, 125–26, 194

R

radar technology, 25

reactive oxygen species (ROS), 36, 86, 90, 205, 225, 231

receptors

  mu-opioid, 111

red light

  benefit of, 39

  bio-stimulatory effects of, 22

red light exposure

  effect on fat oxidation, 147

Red light therapy, 4

  activates fibroblasts, 77

  Alzheimer's disease, 105

  augment testosterone production, 172

  augment testosterone production, 173

  benefits of, 6, 23, 41, 59, 64

  effect on cognitive function, 6

  environmental factors that impact, 244

  for anti-aging, 75

  for men's hormonal health, 172

  impact on carpal tunnel syndrome, 178

  improve cognitive function, 105, 177

  improve mitochondrial function, 86

  in athletic performance, 138

in brain health, 34

on depression, 6

on men's hormonal health, 173

on mental health, 6

on moenoposal symptoms, 168

on stress reduction, 59

on thermogenesis, 147

on weight loss, 145

prevent cellular damage, 106

treatments in aesthetics, 50

Red Light Therapy

benefits of, 142

Red light therapy devices

benefits of LED-based, 68

hybrid, 66

Laser-based, 66

LED-based, 25, 66

respiratory system, 99

RLT. *See* Red light therapy

rosacea, 78

chronic, 123

S

Seasonal Affective Disorder (SAD), 184

seborrheic dermatitis, 80

sebum, 80

regulation, 80

sebum production

RLT in, 124

semiconductor lasers, 66

skin fibroblasts, 95, 204

smallpox

   Red light therapy in treatment of, 52

smart drugs. *See* nootropics

Southern blot, 203

sports medicine

   Red light therapy in, 114

State-Trait Anxiety Inventory (STAI), 59

stress hormone. *See* cortisol

stress management, 242

stress reduction

   techniques, 212

stroke, 185

sunlight

   power of, 15

   use of, 16

superoxide dismutase (SOD), 123

supplements, antioxidant, 244

T

T cells, 214

T lymphocytes. *See* T cells

telomere damage, effects of RLT on, 204

telomere integrity, 203

telomeres, 203, 206, 210

Temporomandibular Disorder (TMD), 109

testosterone, 165, 171

thermogenesis, 147–48

thiobarbituric acid reactive substances (TBARS), 160

tissue damage, 24, 110, 123, 129

tissue oxygenation, 74, 112

total antioxidant capacity (TAC), 160

Townes, Charles, 25

traditional Chinese Medicine, 16

traditional treatments, 52

   for arthritis, 193

   for IBD, 194

traumatic brain injuries (TBIs), 30, 259

Trifecta Light Bed, 69, 250

   and skincare routine, 121

   benefit of, 28

   on inflammation, 200

   on joint mobility, 161

tuberculosis, 16

tuberculosis bacteria, 18

type 2 diabetes, 146, 189, 191, 202

U

Ultraviolet (UV) radiation, 204, 245

ultraviolet (UV) rays, 18

uncoupling proteins (UCPs), 104

V

vascular endothelial growth factor (VEGF), 81

Venier, Leanne, 3

visual analog scale (VAS), 64, 158

vitamins, 235

W

wavelengths of light
  dermal penetration by, *43*
weight loss, 60, 141
Whelan, Harry, 23
white blood cells. *See* leukocytes
Wunsch, Alexander, 63

Printed in Great Britain
by Amazon

29561119R00159